D0724492

Brain Injury
Rewiring

MARGATE CITY PUBLIC LIBRARY

8100 ATLANTIC AVENUE

MARGATE CITY, NJ 08402

(609) 822-4700

www.margatelibrary.org

1. Most items may be checked out for two weeks and renewed for the same period. Additional restrictions may apply to high-demand items.

2. A fine is charged for each day material is not returned according to the above rule. No material will be issued to any person incurring such a fine until it has been paid.

3. All damage to material beyond reasonable wear and all losses shall be paid for.

4. Each borrower is responsible for all items checked out on his/her library card and for all fines accruing on the same.

OCT   2013 DEMCO

AN IDYLL ARBOR PERSONAL HEALTH BOOK

Brain Injury Rewiring
for Survivors

A Lifeline to New Connections

Carolyn E. Dolen, MA

Foreword by Christine A. Baser, PhD

Idyll Arbor

Idyll Arbor, Inc.

39129 264th Ave SE, Enumclaw, WA 98022 (360) 825-7797

Idyll Arbor, Inc. Editor: Thomas M. Blaschko
Back cover photograph: Don Anderson

© Copyright 2010, Carolyn E. Dolen. All rights reserved. No part of this book may be reproduced, stored in a retrieval system, or transcribed, in any form or by any means — electronic, mechanical, photocopying, recording, or otherwise — without the prior written permission of the publisher.

To the best of our knowledge, the information and recommendations of this book reflect currently accepted practice. Nevertheless, they cannot be considered absolute and universal. Recommendations for a particular person must be considered in light of the person's needs and condition. The author and publisher disclaim responsibility for any adverse effects resulting directly or indirectly from the suggested therapy practices, from any undetected errors, or from the reader's misunderstanding of the text.

Library of Congress Cataloging-in-Publication Data

Dolen, Carolyn E., 1946-
  Brain injury rewiring for survivors : a lifeline to new connections / Carolyn E. Dolen ; foreword by Christine A. Baser.
    p. cm.
  "An Idyll Arbor Personal Health Book."
  Includes bibliographical references and index.
  ISBN 978-1-882883-59-2 (alk. paper)
  1. Brain damage--Patients--Rehabilitation. I. Title.
  RC387.5.D65 2010
  617.4'810443--dc22

                                                    2009021783

ISBN 9781882883592

To all survivors

That we may be all we can be.
That our climbs be shared,
That our packs be light,
That our eyes be clear,
And that the vistas be near.

To those who say "You can't,"
Show them you can.
To those who say "You won't,"
Show them you will.

And to those who ask you how —
Just show them.

Contents

Foreword

The brain is a mysterious and wondrous thing: three pounds of jelly-like matter that determines who we are, what we think, how we feel, and how we live in the world. Writing about the brain in an intelligent, cogent, and helpful way is even more wondrous, and that is what Carolyn Dolen has done.

Providing us with two volumes, *Brain Injury Rewiring for Survivors* and *Brain Injury Rewiring for Loved Ones*, is an accomplishment that speaks not only to Carolyn's passion for teaching and sharing, but also her compassion for anyone who has faced life on terms they didn't expect, ask for, or want. During my career as a neuropsychologist I have often wished for a book like *Brain Injury Rewiring* to provide my patients the answers they seek and the inspiration to continue their own journeys.

I remember when Carolyn began the project of *Brain Injury Rewiring*, and while I was amazed at her dedication, I did doubt that she could be so persistent as to compose, rewrite, and edit this volume again and again until it was done. I shouldn't have doubted her determination for this labor of love! Persist Carolyn did, and she has now provided us not only with terrific information and resources, but insight and understanding about the trials and triumphs of traumatic brain injury recovery.

It is fitting that *Brain Injury Rewiring* places Spiritual Rewiring at the front end. If you are reading this, you are likely a "seeker," someone trying to find and connect with whatever lies beyond what you already know. Starting from a spiritual place or "heart center" recognizes that being brain injured is not who a person is; it is their soul that comes closest to revealing their true self. Harmony, new horizons, and heart can be found by any who seek it.

As a neuropsychologist, I relate well to the Cognitive Rewiring chapter. There are many activities that can help retrain cognitive functioning, at any recovery stage. I have found that young survivors tend to embrace technological aids with ease, are still familiar with the learning process, and accept the role of "student" to the therapist's "teacher." They are not as firmly established in their habits and roles, and therefore approach cognitive rehab with less trepidation. Older survivors, more established in a role or life routine, may resist doing things differently than they did before their injury, struggling to accept that a new approach doesn't diminish them. However, older survivors often have the benefit of life experience and prior learning that facilitate cognitive rehab. As Carolyn points out, each person will have a different blueprint of recovery. While cognitive rehabilitation may employ similar learning principles with different survivors, the specific functions focused upon and the amount of compensation versus retraining will vary from person to person.

Emotional rewiring may be the least understood of all. We know the prevalence of typical psychiatric disorders that follow a brain injury and we know that emotional distress is a predictable secondary consequence of trauma and loss. However, we are only beginning to clearly understand how various emotions influence our thoughts and our thoughts affect our emotions. Add to that a brain that sometimes processes information accurately and sometimes does not, and it makes for unpredictable behavior. Many survivors feel emotions more deeply and are easily overwhelmed by emotion, particularly in the early stages after injury. They must relearn how to regulate emotions and control behavior so they are not subject to the strong pull of feelings like a runaway train. In most cases, initial heightened emotional sensitivity smoothes out over time, and residual sentimentality can be channeled into a greater appreciation for life. As you read the Emotional Rewiring chapter, be kind to yourself, non-judgmental, for any of the emotional traumas that still exist.

With her "tell-it-like-it-is" style, Carolyn outlines all the major traditional therapies, and some increasingly popular alternative therapies, in the Body-Mind Rewiring and Mind-Body-Spirit Rewiring chapters. Since there is no one health care specialty that can provide all things to all people, Carolyn wisely emphasizes how to find and keep a good health care team. As the practice of health care evolves, it departs more and more from the days of Marcus Welby, MD or long visits with the familiar family doctor. Each survivor must learn the tools of self-advocacy in order to receive the best care. Carolyn not only provides wonderful descriptions of therapies, but also offers many tips on how to communicate your needs to health care professionals.

The most surprising thing to me about *Brain Injury Rewiring for Survivors* is that Carolyn kept the Nutritional Rewiring and Physical Rewiring chapters to 73 pages! Her editor must have had a hand in that. Healing nutrition has been a mainstay for Carolyn and no doubt contributes greatly to her zest for life. If you wonder why a chapter on nutrition is in a book about brain injury, then you are missing one of the primary take-home messages of this book... your whole self is involved in the healing process. If any part of you is "out of whack," then your healing will be harder to accomplish and take longer.

You will probably detect the former physical education teacher in the Nutritional and Physical Rewiring chapters. You can just picture the food pyramid, nutritional labels, and calipers being offered to all willing students. Seriously though, we can all benefit from Carolyn's experience and knowledge, as she truly "walks the walk" when it comes to nutrition and physical well-being. Scientific studies are showing that the benefits of exercise extend far beyond the physical body, to cognitive and emotional well-being. Most people recognize that nutrition and exercise will create a stronger and more willing body, but the positive impact upon the mind is sorely underestimated. If you haven't already discovered this for yourself, *Brain Injury Rewiring for Survivors* can explain it and show you the way to becoming active and vital.

Sigmund Freud claimed that "love and work are the cornerstones of our humanness." If you are fortunate enough to achieve a good physical, cognitive, and emotional recovery, you might believe that your healing is complete. On the contrary, optimal healing includes a good quality of life, and that means being in the world in a meaningful way. The Social Rewiring and Vocational Rewiring chapters address the biggest challenges a brain injury survivor has to face — *"How will I be received and how do I pull my own weight in the world?"* While gainful employment is not possible for some survivors, I have observed that all survivors want a connection with other people and want to spend time doing something socially worthwhile or personally satisfying. Although finances obviously motivate people to return to work, we see our true selves through what we do and how we spend our time. Carolyn makes it easier to navigate the confusing world of social relationships, financial support, and vocational re-entry. The acronym SAFER, used throughout this book, is applied particularly well to the topics of social and vocational rewiring.

The scientific literature has a great deal to say about the role of awareness in brain injury recovery. In the patients I have worked with over the years I have found that awareness characterizes successful survivors: awareness of themselves, their circumstances, and their options. They don't just wait and then react. They actively size things up and figure out their place in the scheme of things. They are aware of what is or is not working for them.

Brain Injury Rewiring for Survivors is a terrific tool for increasing awareness. Carolyn has posed thoughtful and revealing questions and created a template for staying open and aware. If you read and use *Brain Injury Rewiring for Survivors* as the guide it was meant to be, then you will undoubtedly improve your awareness and contribute to your success.

Read. Begin. Heal.

— Christine A. Baser, PhD
Neuropsychologist
Carlsbad, California
May 2009

Acknowledgements

To rewire body, mind, and spirit after a brain injury requires lots of helpers (as described in Chapter Two). Here I will endeavor to thank all of the many angels whom God sent to me. More than thirty years have elapsed since I started this journey, and someone may be inadvertently omitted, despite God's efforts to awaken me at 5 AM with names on the brain! Please forgive me if I miss one of you. You all really did help, and survivors sometimes don't remember everything, as most of you undoubtedly already know.

This list starts with my best friend since 1976, Marlys Henke, who offered her hearth, as well as her heart, mind, and pocketbook many times during the course of our cross-country friendship. It all began with a chance encounter on our first day of teachers' meetings at Highland Park Junior High in St. Paul, Minnesota. I asked her to join several of us at lunch. Funny how it's all worked out. She invited me to her Methodist Church home, affiliated with United Ministries in Higher Education (UMHE), located on the University of Minnesota campus. This church connection also enriched our friendship. Indeed, God works in mysterious ways.

Another angel was my childhood friend, Louise Lentz, who nourished me and visited me, even in locked wards and other undesirable places, just because I needed her. Friends from Johnson High School, like Mike Kluznik, and St. Olaf College alum Ann Jorstad stuck with me through many travails and helped me to remember that I was still lovable and fun. So did Pat Marshall, a dear friend since the 1980s from my San Diego days.

"Body and spirit" professionals who were especially helpful fit into the "Friends" category because the best ones acted as professionals who were friends. My willpower alone would not have gotten me up the rehab mountain. I needed the loving persistence — and wisdom — of these special people, who believed, respected, and cared.

The first of these is DJ (Dale Johnson, PhD of El Paso, Texas), who unfortunately is not physically alive to see my current status on the mountain, but I know that he knows where I am. Without DJ, I'd probably still be kicking holes in desks, punching holes in walls, screaming, crying, and cutting and burning my arm — or in some state mental hospital, homeless, or dead. Until his death in 1991, DJ visited, called, and wrote to ensure my psyche stayed on course.

Significant professionals in the 1980s include Liana Beckett, an MFCC intern at the UCSD Gifford Clinic, who continued to help me sort out the puzzle, and Mary-Alice Isenhart, PhD, who taught me that it is okay to be a strong woman. My 1990s team starts with Christine Baser, PhD, who lovingly empowered me to make significant changes in a short amount of time. Dr. Baser referred me to Daniel Gardner, MD, who treated me with respect, which enabled me to trust a male psychiatrist, even with a nineteen-year history of failure, both with MDs and drugs. Another Dr. Baser referral, Kent Bennington, PhD, used Eye Movement Desensitization and Reprocessing (EMDR), to end my irrational fears relative to the trauma of a post-injury sexual assault in 1976 and the various associated fears from the auto accident that necessitated this long climb.

Nathan Zasler, MD, most assuredly belongs on this list, not only for his brain injury treatment guidance, suggesting the Brain Tuner that replaced Prozac, but also the faithful mentoring that began in January, 1995. Dr Z (as I call him) provided the first review of *Brain Injury Rewiring*, a critique that led to my first contract. Survivors everywhere thank you, Dr. Zasler, for igniting *Brain Injury Rewiring*!

While I've needed less care since 1999, angels who helped heal wounds included Margaret November, MD, who noticed my occasional twitching, heretofore unrecognized, and prescribed Neurontin, which I can also use if/when I feel depressed or anxious. (The grey and cold winters still plague me.) Then in 2008 when I experienced PTSD from two rear-end collisions in a year, I sought an EMDR practitioner because it worked so well previously. Fortunately, I found my current on-call angel, Kay Emerick, PhD, with whom I immediately connected. She, like the other best helpers, maintained eye contact, took few notes, and seemed to actually like me — even expressing it! Other current loving members of my health care team include acupuncturist Mike Long, chiropractor Robert Cocain, DC, and Gulnar Poorsattar, MD. I feel very blessed!

To heal my spirit, I looked to the church, which lightened my load on many occasions. Early on, in 1976-78, it was Bill Mate, minister at UMHE, who patiently provided weekly counseling when no other services could or would handle my morass of problems. As part of the University outreach program, Bill, a noted writer, led a weekly group on writing exercises that ventured into safe areas and provided a wonderful escape route for me.

Following Bill in 1978 was a minister in El Paso, Texas. She and her family took me in after the YWCA called with a desperate plea for housing for a woman with a disabled vehicle, who was far from home — and without funds. This kind family offered a sanctuary for me for several weeks, and the Catholic Church accepted me in worship, even without nice clothes. Another early angel was the tow truck driver in Van Horn, Texas, who invited me to stay with him and his other three roommates (without disturbing me!) because I had no money and no place to go after the engine of my MG blew up in the Van Horn Mountains on my way from Minnesota to California in 1980. Thank you, too, for towing my MG to El Paso out of the goodness of your heart.

During my El Paso stay, a call from a friend brought me to New York City, where I reveled in the pomp and ceremony of St. Patrick's Cathedral. The ritual of the mass calmed my brain and the warmth and light of the votive candles brought me closer to the higher power who could help me. Thank you to the people who paid for the many candles I lit each week.

In the winter of 1980 I finally made it to San Diego (my initial destination when I set out from St. Paul, Minnesota, that cold winter day in 1978). My newly repaired MG brought me to Mission Beach. At St. Brigid's Catholic Church in nearby Pacific Beach, Father Lloyd and Father Richard welcomed me and introduced me to other young adults in a wonderful folk singing group. One of those members, Vanessa Puniak, remains a friend today. I remember that once Father Richard even dug unto his pockets for a $100 bill to pay for my car insurance. There, too, I met Beth Le Friant, who allowed me to camp out on her living room floor for a while. Then Northminster Presbyterian briefly became my church home; Bobbie McKee is still a friend today from that connection.

After I moved north to Encinitas, I was led to Christ Presbyterian Church of Rancho La Costa where I was first warmly welcomed by Interim Pastor Steve Jenks and Associate Pastor Ed Reynolds, PhD, and then later by Pastor Doug Kelly. I loved singing in the choir under the loving and forgiving leadership of Bergitta Brice and teaching Sunday school. It was so much fun to teach kids again! I still fondly remember Courtney and April Allen; the Artz girls: Erin, Kylie, and Aubrey; Laura and Megan Jones; Teddy Minner; and Allison and Martha Wright, who all ably assisted my teaching and didn't mind my non-adult behavior. There I was blessed with loving kindnesses especially by Dixie Jacobson and the Banes, Billings, Hayens, McCarters, Petersons, Wings; and dear, sweet MaryAnn Christ, who befriended me through all sorts of trials, took me to dinner, briefly housed me, walked with me on the beach, and listened and loved me. Another member, computer genius Reese Brown, volunteered to format and print the very first edition of *Brain Injury Rewiring* — all 86-pages! Thank you and bless you all!

Then the Episcopal Church — and more healing music — called me, first to St. Andrew's in Encinitas, then to St. Michael's in Carlsbad, and finally to St. Paul's Episcopal in Ventura and my beloved and supportive priest, Father Jerry Kahler. There was a brief interim stop at First Presbyterian in Santa Barbara, when I lived in my office (thank you to the lessee who kindly allowed me to sublet and sleep on the floor, while ignoring security reports!). Speaking of sleeping, without the Ventura Housing Authority and the Section 8 Program, I'd be homeless.

For brain rewiring, I first turned to school, starting with a study skills class and a reading improvement class way back in 1976. Building on my strengths is what the most notable professors did in my many ventures into the academic world. When my confidence allowed it, I began another graduate school program in counseling in the fall of 1977 at nearby University of Wisconsin at River Falls (UWRF). There I interacted with more wonderful, loving people.

One of my first post-injury professors, Dr. Vanetta Ogland, taught a psychology class entitled "Exceptional Children." After our first test, when I reported that I had over-studied, she responded, "All good students do." This was the very first time since the accident that I recall anyone ever telling me that I was good at anything. So I worked my tail off, loved her class, and even earned an A! She was the first one to call my writing "haunting," after she read one of my pieces about "The Boy from Avreyon," the story of the boy who lived in the wild and then was "saved" by some townspeople. (She noted my line "and he never smiled again.").

Also significant at UWRF was Bill Romoser, PhD, statistics professor, whose love for aphorisms kept me going ("It's tough to fly with eagles when you work for turkeys," and "Don't let the bastards get you down." (He said this in Latin to be PC, but I don't remember it.) Another was Counselor John Hamann, PhD, who took on the challenge of working with my psyche. John used my intellect and stubbornness to advantage, challenging me to overcome the demons. Without enough weapons, I couldn't yet, but his assistant, Joann introduced me to the desensitization techniques that would be very useful in many areas throughout my journey.

There were also special professors at Cal State Dominguez Hills, where I earned my first MA in Special Education in 1986. My adviser, Karl Skindrud, PhD, kindly helped me finish the program in ten months, while teaching full-time, even though when I told him my plan at our initial meeting, he said, "No one has ever done that." (I probably said, "Watch me," or something equally diplomatic.) Intellectual stimulation and emotional support in that program was provided by Judith Jackson, PhD, the language professor who actually made studying speech interesting.

After returning to San Diego and briefly teaching, I studied at San Diego State University from 1988-91. Special professors in the Physical Education Department (now known as Exercise Science) included Pete Aufsesser, PhD; Peggy Lasko-McCarthy, PhD; Tom McKenzie, PhD; and department chair, Rob Carlson, PhD. Another Midwest refugee, Pat Patterson, PhD, who played the role of active guardian angel during my coursework, thesis work, and extensions, voluntarily chaired my thesis committee and worked with me weekly for nine months to restore my writing skills, develop a researcher's questioning mind, and befriend me generally. Uncannily, Pat could act knowledgeably, yet defer to me as the brain injury expert and allow me to develop the topic.

During my thirty-plus-year journey, I could always rely on physical activity to produce joy. And, while I've lifted weights in many different gyms across the country, my favorite indoor "fitness home" is the Ventura Family YMCA. The excitement that results from a wide diversity of ages is so refreshing. Not only am I thankful for the scholarship that allows me to be a member, but also for the accepting and happy feeling that permeates the facility. I don't mind that I'm often the only female in the free weight room either! Yoga Jones is my other indoor haven from stress.

Finally, I am very grateful to my brilliant and accommodating friends who supported my efforts and edited one or many chapters, starting again with Marlys Henke. Thank you, too, to my talented photographer, Don Anderson (with three PhDs!) and his able assistants, Joan Anderson and Susan Abrams, who are members of St. Paul's in Ventura. Actually, my entire church family, especially Kay Armstrong and the Leahys, deserve a huge thank you for supporting *Brain Injury Rewiring* and me for the past nine years! Many editors are church friends, including: Ralph Armstrong, MD, Bill Knutson, Dev Leahy (DevL), Larry Meyers, MD, and Jennie Whaley. Valuable help in dissecting dozens of research studies was provided by Diane Rennell, PhD, whom I met while ushering in Ventura. Thanks also to Mark Ylvisaker, PhD, who communicated with me for years despite battling melanoma; Rob Rich, DC, and John Dupler, PhD, for their chapter contributions; and early editors, Christine Baser, PhD, and Dan Gardner, MD, who labored over long chapters. For igniting the *Brain Injury Rewiring* spark, I'm indebted to the San Diego Brain Injury Foundation (SDBIF) for funding my initial thesis research and its former president Ron Ruff, PhD, for supporting it. Lastly, *Brain Injury Rewiring* would not even exist as a "New Connection" if not for the courage of Tom Blaschko of Idyll Arbor who persevered with me for five years from contract to final product. No doubt there were a few (or many) times he wondered about his own sanity during this adventure!

Throughout this thirty-plus-year journey, many other angels entered my life and offered their hearts, minds, backs, and, a few, even their pocketbooks, to lessen my load and lift me to the ledges beyond my reach. *Brain Injury Rewiring* is my thanks to you generous souls for your small and large acts of kindness. Know that others will reach the top because you first helped me. Bless you one and all!

Introduction

Life is a one-way street. No matter how many
detours you take, none of them leads back.
And once you know and accept that, life
becomes much simpler. Because then you
know you must do the best you can with what
you have and what you are and what you have
become.

— Isabel Moore

Brain Injury Rewiring for Survivors: A Lifeline to New Connections is
my gift of a helping hand to all who seek one in our climb up the
recovery mountain. I offer my hand and ask that you, in turn, give yours
to others, so that no one feels that no one cares.

From my experience as a survivor, I will offer you ideas about how
to heal your body, mind, and spirit as you make new connections to
yourself and to others so that you can successfully reenter your
community and resume productive activity.

I share my journey with you — and dare you to "Just Do It!" too —
go over, under, around, or through those obstacles in your path!

Brain Injury Rewiring for Survivors: A Lifeline to New Connections
is half of a two-part set — *Brain Injury Rewiring for Loved Ones: a
Lifeline to New Connections* is my gift to your loved ones. My books can
help all of you learn how to make new connections as you — the
survivor — rewire your brain. I prove that recovery is possible — with a
spark and some hot wires! Get charged!

1
Recollections of *the* Day

In the middle of the journey of our life, I came to myself in a dark wood where the straight path was lost.

— Dante

Old Highway 12, Inver Grove Heights, Minnesota
January 10, 1976, 11:37 AM

It happened on a snowy, blowy, winter day in Minnesota over three decades ago. As my mind flashed back to the ski lesson and ahead to seeing Hank, the friendly flurries of the morning gradually changed to gusts, and then to whiteout, obscuring the lane lines on Old Highway 12.

Soon the surface itself became almost invisible and I couldn't see if there even was a road! Every cell of my being focused on navigating my cherry-red MG Midget out of the turmoil of the storm and into the haven of my garage, just a few miles away.

Then, as snow blanketed the pavement and left me blizzard-blind, it happened — crash! My brain cannot remember and my soul cannot forget the collision. This is the conversation I had with myself that day:

"Boy, do I love to ski! It reminds me of cycling. Skis glide without effort, as I fly down hills, wind in my face, free — free to be. Actually, it's just great to be outside, exercising. I feel so alive, whole, happy — just being outdoors.

3

It's so unlike working at the hobby shop. What a bore! Hmmm, maybe I should call personnel on Monday and try teaching again; it sure wouldn't be boring. I'm just on extended sick leave, anyway.

Boy! Do I ever miss my old teaching job! I probably wouldn't have ulcers if I were still there. Darn it! What a great staff! We all really cared about one another, unlike that last place. What a switch! Still, despite no adult friends there, I liked most of the kids and even though the teaching wasn't as fun, the coaching, as always, was worth it. And working with the kids usually took my mind off the divorce.

God! I never thought divorce would be so awful, so lonely, so sad. But I just didn't like where our marriage was going and he refused to go to therapy with me. I suppose he thought he'd be outnumbered, me in a graduate program in counseling and all. I'm so sorry he didn't want to save it, not to mention shocked. I'll really miss his mother. God, I love her. I hope we can still be friends.

Well, my mother was right about John. I hate it when she's right! Sure am glad to have Hank in my life, but when is he going to be free? I guess I should be happy just to share what time we have. Can't wait to see him! All I have to do is watch for my exit. I'm almost there.

Okay, you're close. All you have to do is stay on the road. Find the exit. Are you in the right lane? Oops, better be sure. Go slowly, stay on the road."

That's all I remember. Now I am a survivor: someone who lived through an accident that caused a brain injury.

The Pre-Injury Person: Similarities Survivors Share

Many survivors and family members will recognize my chaotic life was similar to their own experiences. Although many of us would prefer to "idealize the deceased" — a psychological term for describing the pre-injury person as nearly perfect — research suggests that many survivors' lives immediately before the injury were lives of turbulence, disorder, and overwhelming risk-taking behavior.

That survivors share many similarities is well known: Those under age 30 incur 70% of all injuries, with males two to three times more likely to be involved than females. Survivors are four times more likely to be divorced and are unemployed more often than not. Significantly, nearly 75% of us survived a transport-related accident. Finally, the most significant contributing factor to all accidents is the use of alcohol, although not in my case — it was still morning!

On the spiritual side, if we survivors are honest about our pre-injury lives, there was no apparent life or focus of energy for many of us. The story you are about to read may not fit all survivors. It simply illustrates one kind of chaos — yours may have been different. We all came from different places, worked at different jobs, and may or may not have been in a loving relationship. But one thing we all share: we are now brain-injured, and our lives will never again be the same.

Revealing some of this history may tarnish my girl-next-door image for both old and new friends, but it's the truth — as far as I can remember. Facing that truth is vital for survivors to move past what was, to focus on what is, and what can be.

My Muddled Career and Emotional Life

Pre-injury, my life was a mess! Career, emotional, physical, and spiritual aspects were all in disarray, marked by questionable decisions that were likely influenced by alcohol and mostly prescription drugs — and maybe just a little "herb."

The structure that arises from a stable home and job life began to unravel, starting with a minor accident that resulted in a whiplash injury, for which I received cortisone injections and Valium prescriptions.

Then came the separation from my "until death do us part" husband of five years — a defining crack in my '50s and '60s fairy tale world that advertised: "Get a degree and follow that with an optional career. But be sure to marry, and make a home, and then live happily every after." Couples were supposed to agree on everything, and the fairy tale never told us what to do if incompatibility developed as people grew. After all, did Ozzie and Harriet ever fight?

In addition to the injury and the flaw in the marriage fairy tale, the fatal flaw ultimately proved to be in my workaday fairy tale: my teaching career at a beloved school was over. Reduced enrollment at the junior high where I taught, coached, counseled, and chaired the social committee forced an involuntary transfer.

In two months I lost both the security of a relatively stable home life and a very fulfilling work environment where I was loved, valued, and allowed to grow. This was followed by a bewildering summer filled with long walks and talks with friends that focused on the shock of a failed marriage. Graduate school, poetry workshops, and new friends from those endeavors helped ease the pain, but the summer's culminating move to a tiny apartment seemed to symbolize all that I lost. My new place lacked personality, pool, tennis courts — and my marriage partner. It visibly represented the emptiness that I felt.

The flaw in the fairy tale widened that fall and grew to a chasm when I realized that none of the features of my former beloved school — young, strong, close staff; programs that worked; energy; community support — were present in the new school. Perhaps more importantly, I was not a vital part of it. There was no reason to esteem newcomer me or seek my input. Still reeling from — and barely surviving — the losses, I was unable to find my role in this entrenched system, dashing my hope of a fresh career start.

At this school I met Hank, who pretended to be single, but wasn't, which I learned after I fell in love with him. The typical empty promise to get a divorce "...as soon as..." further disrupted the fairy tale.

Hospitalization for an ulcer attack interrupted this confusing scene, first on a medical floor — then on the psychiatric wing! After a bewildering month, I was released and found a special position at an experimental school offering strong people and energy, but not the structure and belonging I so desperately needed.

After vagabonding between the homes of parents and various friends, I moved back to the same apartment building of my married life, and began the next year at yet another school I didn't like, which had even fewer of the qualities I valued.

Then another hospitalization. This time it was straight to the psychiatric ward — for depression and ulcers again. As part of my treatment plan, doctors recommended I take an extended sick leave from my now very unfulfilling teaching career and work part-time in sales at a nearby hobby shop. This sounded appropriate for two reasons: I was born to sell and the sales job would be less stressful. But it lacked vitality, even at Christmas, and I missed teaching, missed the kids — and missed the feeling of doing something worthwhile.

During this tumultuous year and a half, my support network — parents, family, friends — were still dealing with the fact I was no longer part of a couple — my parents reacted with anger and my friends and family with avoidance. After they initially comforted me, I lost my close circle of loved ones. Most old friends were temporarily out of touch at this time — everyone struggled with their own issues.

My only spiritual life was that found at the end of a bong or in a bottle of Scotch, in bed, or behind the wheel of my cherished red MG Midget. I vaguely remember a bit — maybe a lot — of sexual acting-out. Physically, I was not able to consistently exercise. Still suffering with whiplash from two minor accidents — before the MG — I took Valium at will and often washed it down with an alcoholic beverage while out socializing. Besides this self-medication, I randomly took other drugs that doctors prescribed for depression. Did I mention a certain fondness for marijuana in a wine-filled bong?

The pre-injury portrait you've just read paints a life in turmoil, to be sure. Career and marriage lost, our girl-next-door was struggling — and losing. Although my memory is somewhat cloudy, it's likely that I simply do not recall other disturbing events, probably in an unconscious attempt to maintain some semblance of dignity — I ask your understanding for that. But even with no other contributing factors, you get the picture. It is not surprising that I was an accident waiting to happen. I do vividly remember the following scene at the hospital — terror does that.

After the Injury, Ramsey Medical Center St. Paul, Minnesota January 10, 1976, 6:11 PM

Where am I? Why is everything dark? Hank and I were supposed to meet at noon. What are my parents doing here, standing over by that window? My mother looks worried. She's wearing that frown and my father looks distressed — I guess. I've never seen that look on his face before. It's sort of mad and sad at the same time.

Oh, God! What's the matter with me? Why can't I move? Why am I strapped down? Why does my head hurt? Why does everything hurt? Why can't I talk? Am I dead? Where am I? Why am I in this gown, in this bed, in this strange, dark room? Why are my parents looking at me like that?

I want to say, "Hi!" and smile, so my mother will stop frowning — but I can't, so I moan. They look at me and Mom says, "Honey, you're in the hospital and you had a bad car accident, but the doctor says you'll be fine."

Oh God, No! Not my MG — my precious MG — not my MG!

That's all I remember. That — and the absolute terror of not being able to speak.

End of Day 1

Beginning of the climb — the endless climb — the climb that demands your all — the climb that either kills you or makes you strong.

2
Climbing the Mountain

This time it's make or break. All senses concentrate. He knows that's what it takes. For a victory. Only the strongest survive. No room for compromise. He races with the time. And his own mortality. Some people don't know how to give in. You knock 'em down. They just pick themselves up again. And all they got is. Willpower. To make a dream come true. Don't underestimate willpower. It can move a mountain or two.

— G. Lyle, T. Britten

The crash forever changed my concentration — from navigating my beloved MG to navigating myself through the windy, tortuous switchbacks that meander up the mountain of life. I describe my more than 30-year ascent in the following story, where an avalanche substitutes for the car crash.

Today, my climb up the mountain continues, on the surface not all that different from others navigating through the ordinary switchbacks of their lives. But after an avalanche interrupted my previous expedition, careening me onto a rocky ledge, several things do distinguish me from my fellow travelers. Now my brain needs direct commands and half of my body wants to rest while the other half works. And although I look fine, neither my repaired equipment nor my old clothes seem to fit. Funny how no one else notices.

Other members of my hiking party move faster than I. They question my slow pace; I look like I'm in shape for this journey, except for a few cuts and bruises.

It's at times like these that I wish for a defining scar of some sort, a visible sign of my limits, like a big "HI" for "head-injured" prominently displayed on my forehead. Then maybe people would give me a break. And I could give myself a break. But they'd probably see it as a greeting and say, "Hi!" — or ask for an explanation that could lead me to an outburst, which would just make everything worse. As it is, I look fine.

No one gives me credit for surviving the near-fatal avalanche, rehabilitating myself, and setting out on yet another climb. What does happen, however, is that other hikers frequently nag me to move faster and tell me to lighten my load if I can't make it. They offer suggestions that begin with "Why don't you just ..." and say, "You don't look disabled to me." Funny how no one asks me if I have a problem.

Exasperated at my halting steps, one of the leaders places an extra sun visor on my head, convinced that the bright sun is slowing my progress. But the hat slips down my sweaty forehead, covers my good eye, and I'd have to drop the lifeline to fix it. Now the only visible direction is down, the crooked hat masks my tears, and I struggle even more. Funny how no one sees this.

Some fellow climbers doubt my efforts and challenge my courage. "What's the matter, why can't you keep up? My pack is bigger than yours. You said you were a tough athlete." This is followed by more "Why don't you just ..." suggestions with variations on the "Try a little harder!" theme. Oh, I wish I had that scar and didn't look so fine. But still, it's funny how no one tries to understand.

The other hikers offer many suggestions except for the one that would help — offering to carry part of my load. Perhaps because each pack has been custom-designed, no one wants to take part of my pack's weight, create an imbalance, and jeopardize his own success. Funny about that.

Everyone tells me how much easier it would be if I had been able to save my original equipment. No kidding. This is followed by marveling at how lucky I was to survive with so little damage and how good I look. Sporting a very large scar increases in appeal by the minute. Then maybe they'd commend me for my efforts — perhaps even ask how to help me.

As it is, as they continue their climbs, they laugh at the repaired gear that hasn't adjusted to my new shape. I force a smile to avoid the extra burden of an outburst, try to hold back my tears, and talk to God and to myself.

"Remember, 'Act as if' — as if you're not weak, not inadequate, as if you can do it." I stumble on, but without laughing. It's not funny.

Maybe they forget that I, too, loved my original form-fitting pack. I need to remember that they mean well, and that at least we're still on the journey together. After all, they haven't asked me to leave their group — yet. I hope they remember that I'm doing the best I can. Funny how no one offers to change places with me. And I don't even have a scar. *"It could be worse. I could be falling or stuck at the bottom or alone."*

Suddenly, there's a shelf and a hand reaches down to help pull me up. The sun and the other hikers warmly greet me. My tears are over, for now, replaced by a smile and a thank-you. The next ledge is in view and the mountaintop — shrouded by clouds since the beginning of the climb — actually looks reachable. Funny about that.

My Three Helping Hands

Most survivors likely will empathize with this story — and also understand that everyone carries a loaded backpack. Hopefully, most loved ones and professionals will help to carry part of our load. Indeed, what we all really need to climb the mountain is a helping hand.

To explain why I now mostly peer down at the vista below me instead of being mired in the muck at the bottom or marooned on an obscure ledge on the mountainside, I can think of three reasons:

- God, church, and my religious family — my spiritual life.
- Willpower, hard work, and achievable goals — my values, beliefs, and attitudes.
- Friends and family — my support system.

All of these are interdependent, e.g., many friends are from my religious family — and none of them could carry the extra load alone.

Even with God on my side, if there were no God's helpers or no Minnesota work ethic, my journey would likely have ended long ago. For any significant, lasting progress to occur I still need them all.

A good example of all my helpers working together followed my running a 5K race, attended by members of my adopted San Diego family. A 20-foot high rock-climbing wall attracted the teenager in our family. Because there would be over an hour's wait, I agreed to stand in the long line with him. As we stood there, I noticed that most of the other climbers were between 10 and 40 years younger than I. Two women only a decade or so younger cajoled me into climbing, too. They even requested that I climb first since I had run the race and looked to be in shape.

My anxiety increased as we neared the wall. Questions peppered my mind: *"Where are they placing their limbs to successfully climb? What doesn't work? How did that kid race up the wall so fast? Why doesn't anyone here look remotely close to my age? Why am I so anxious — don't I always say I love to try new things — am I becoming conservative? What would be the worst thing that could happen?"*

The teenager was next and quickly scampered to the top. It was my turn. *"OK, use the holds that the others did. Good! Hands and feet are in place. Oops, now what?"* After one more move, my face nearly touched the wall, every muscle in my body was tense, I was stretched to the limit — and I was stuck.

Seeing the panicked look on my face, family members loudly cheered. As this power surged through me, I scanned the wall for places to move to. Then — luckily — the staff person advised me where to place my left foot. *"Way over there?"* I said to myself. It seemed too far to stretch, but I didn't have another alternative, so attempted the reach — and happily found myself stretching farther than I ever imagined I could!

The rest of the climb was easy, and I reached the top to ring the bell and cheer loudly. *"Wow! After that one obstacle, it was easy to succeed!"* Thanks to all the helpers, I made it — my first wall-climbing experience was a success!

This rock-climbing wall is a metaphor for survivors climbing the recovery mountain: if we stretch farther than we think we can, we can achieve; if we prepare, we can succeed; if at first we don't succeed, try,

try again. Sometimes we may need to just have faith that help is there, even if we cannot see it. The obstacle needn't defeat us just because it looks impassable. We need all of our helpers to work at the same time in order to succeed.

My teenage friend and I moved on to the more advanced wall with confidence. There we were able to place our hands in holds that we could not see after the helpers assured us those were the ones we

> The distance doesn't matter; only the first step is difficult.
> — Mme. du Deffand

needed. We believed them because they had been correct earlier and there appeared to be no other holds that would work anyway. In fact, all the crevices seemed to shrink as we reached them! Thanks to all working together, we climbed up this wall faster than the first and easier one, clanged the bell, and cheered.

Can survivors use my experience on their mountain climbs? Will others see my success and gain enough courage to either start their climbs or continue their journeys with more resolve and confidence? That's my hope.

December 1978 — and the rest of my life

I'll never forget my prognosis after I was injured in 1976: "suicide or psych ward." I remember being both surprised and shocked by what they said. Here I was, a schoolteacher, someone who believed in the power of education to change lives, and they wrote me off! Not only did I wonder what those %?$*&#! were on, but it motivated me to prove them wrong! And it still does — this is why I am writing this book!

Just because I seemed to favor both the excitement of driving an MG and occasionally the security of the psychiatric hospital didn't necessarily make me suicidal and schizophrenic! I simply needed to find my purpose and focus again — to start over — following a period of living on the edge, walking with the devil, and feeling adrift.

After my world blew up, I needed to replace it — with something better! My two years of trauma — including failed suicide attempts — only reaffirmed my belief that, as my childhood friend Louise said,

"You're here for a reason, Carolyn." My mission was to find that purpose before my capabilities were lessened any more.

To prepare for any mission, an inventory needs to be taken: What do I have? What do I need? Where am I going? What do I seek?

Before I could "go with God," I needed to see my way through a dilemma: if God doesn't make junk, why do I feel like it? A typical God response — unpredictable and provocative — arrived at a freeway exit stoplight:

"Child, you were chosen, not discarded. And I chose you because you are strong. Many others are not as strong as you, so you need to help them to carry their load — and I will help you to carry yours. Remember, Jesus already took the big rap. You don't need to carry all of it, too. I'm not asking you to do that. What I am asking is for you to be the best you that you can be. And, when you feel down, remember how tough you are. It is because you are tough that I ask a bit more of you. I will not ask you to do more than you are able. Just call on me when you feel weak and, together, we will prevail. Just remember to call on me."

I paused. My thinking did a 180° turn — from feeling discarded to feeling chosen. So, that's why all the hell — to prove to myself how strong I was. Then, my first positive self-talk in a long time: "You must be pretty damn tough to withstand all that you have faced. And, you have prevailed!"

After this awakening, I could proceed to answer my mission questions: What do we have? What do we need? Where are we going? Why? What if?

First, what I had: cold Minnesota, with snow, ice, scary roads, and six weeks — maybe — of summer complete with the "State Bird" — the mosquito; Mom and Dad — but they're gone all the time, especially in the winter; Aunt Chelsie, Marlys, Louise, and Mary Ellen; bad memories of accident, rape, and school lay-off; vocational/academic failure, and the cabin.

Second, what I needed: something better. With warm weather, ocean, and freedom from snow and cold and scary roads. A fresh start. A graduate school for social work.

Third, where am I going? Either California or Hawaii is warm and provides both the ocean and appropriate graduate schools.

Fourth, why? What if? I can and I must. It is suicide to stay. I need to be free of the snow, the bad memories. If I don't like it, I can always return. Go now before the worst of the snow and cold. This is reminder enough that I must go or I'll die here, unfulfilled.

So, one cold, snowy, winter day in December of 1978, I left Minnesota. One warm, sunny, winter day in December of 1980, I arrived in the Mission Beach community of San Diego, California. A snowdrift in southern Minnesota waylaid me, and the same Rocky Mountain blizzards that blocked the shortest route led me to my wonderful El Paso shrink DJ. It was a two-year journey — a lifetime of experiences that can be revisited at will.

It wasn't easy or fast. But it did happen and it's still happening. I remember my first race of any kind in twenty years: I cycled thirty miles in just over an hour and a half (1:34) to place second to an All-American triathlete in my over-50 age group in a bicycle road race! My new built-up cycling shoes with special inserts actually provided me with two good legs. The result was a shock — no pain and no flats — and I had not trained! Imagine what will happen when I do! When's the next race?!

My recovery over these past thirty-plus years has, in some ways, been nothing short of a miracle — if the many brushes with death and further injury encountered on this journey are considered. In writing this book, even I am amazed at the outcome after all my adventures!

My Invitation to You

Come with me now, as we climb this mountain together. Let's explore how to mend that equipment and even make our peace with it from time to time. Let's treat those wounds and reduce those stumbles.

> Don't underestimate willpower. It can move a mountain or two.
>   — G. Lyle, T. Britten

Let's reach the top — or at least higher than we thought we could. Let's lighten the loads of our fellow travelers — we know what a difference that can make. Eventually, when we begin to hike more and stumble less, and after we reach a ledge or two, we'll breathe easier. Maybe we'll even enjoy the rest of the climb!

3
Brain Construction and Wiring

Do what you can, with what you have, where you are.

— Theodore Roosevelt

After your injury, you probably seek answers to questions like these: "What happened when my brain was injured?" "How does it repair itself?" "Will I recover?" "What can I do to rewire it?" "How long will it take?"

Keep asking! Learning how your brain works will help your recovery! This chapter summarizes the information found in the *Brain Injury Rewiring for Loved Ones* "Brain Construction and Wiring" chapter. Plus there are some special questions that are here just for you.

Terminology. Discussing brain recovery requires the use of some medical vocabulary that may be unfamiliar to you. Please do not skip over these challenging words! All medical terms are *italicized*, defined in the text, and listed in the index.

With billions of *neurons* (nerve cells in the brain) and astronomical numbers of interconnections between them, we all hold tremendous potential! Yes, even survivors still possess a few billion *neurons* ready and waiting! As a teacher, I

> If ye have faith as a grain of mustard seed … nothing shall be impossible to you.
> — Matthew 17:20

believe that people will make good choices if they are educated. Let's begin the understanding phase of our "brain work."

Injuries, Damage, and Effects

Like a precious castle surrounded by a moat, our brains are well protected. Under the skull, several layers of membranes pad the brain physically. Chemically, a multi-layered barrier surrounds all brain cells. Providing the first wall of defense is the *blood-brain barrier (BBB)*, an intricate network of cells that acts like a filtering system, allowing only selected substances to pass. To process and convey information, our *neurons* communicate much like a telephone system.

What happened when my brain was injured?
A chain reaction of events occurred that changed the balance of the brain chemistry. Even if the area that is damaged is small, the entire brain is affected if the *BBB* has been invaded or broken down.

When the *BBB* is violated, a flood of blood cells and other substances that are toxic to *neurons* fill the cellular spaces reserved for them. Just like other unexpected and unwanted floods, the fluid builds rapidly and the brain swells. This swelling is called *edema*.

Glial cells (non-nerve brain cells) protect *neurons* from the toxins and act like sponges, but they swell too and die when overloaded. No amount of sandbags can stop the flow of this flooded river. The toxic chemicals are re-released into the brain's blood circulation system, thereby damaging or killing more *neurons* and *glial cells* because their membranes are overloaded. This allows highly electrically charged particles called *free radicals* to freely roam and assault brain cells. Brain stability is imperiled and chaos reigns. Every living cell reacts with shock.

The brain tries to fight back and adjust to the invasion. The injured cells do everything in their power to live, but the longer the flood continues, the more damage and functional impairment results. What was a balanced "soup" is now a dangerous soup. Where healthy cells once received proper nourishment and oxygen, the rupture of blood vessels means that the transport system no longer works, so elements critical to survival are unavailable. More cell death occurs.

How does the injury affect my communication system?
Electrical impulses sent from *neuron* to *neuron* are interrupted and signals are incomplete. Portions of the brain may no longer communicate with one another or signals may advance at a much slower speed. Disruptions can involve both processing speed and ability. In the case of a severe injury, some neurons actually die; other neurons may be active, but no longer be as efficient.

To use a computer analogy, when the interruption of activity takes the brain down, it may flash distress signals, produce strange noises and symbols, or simply stop. A single disconnected wire halts all activity and nothing anyone does can fix it until and unless the proper wire is reconnected. Then the computer may need to reprogram all its basic functions. It will not just pick up and carry on as if nothing happened. Although it may have only been bumped, incurring an injury that looked minor, the effect of the shock on the total operation was not minor — it may not even know the date and time anymore.

Tests and Treatments

From blinking lights to beeping machines, you may or may not remember much about the early hours and days in the hospital — except that everything hurt.

I vaguely remember watching the monitor screen with fascination and wondering — during my in-and-out-of-consciousness state — what it was showing. I also recall pleading for water for my parched throat and the nurse only placing a few tiny ice chips on my tongue. Now I know the purpose was to restrict my fluids to reduce brain swelling — but then I was feeling victimized by their stinginess with water.

Recovery/Rewiring Questions

Can my brain ever recover its functions? How does it repair?
Yes! Some improvement can occur even years after injury. While we know that the most rapid recovery from head trauma occurs in the first six months, steady and gradual improvement from severe injuries is often

observed for two years or so after injury, and progress may continue at a slower rate for several more years.

According to Stein, Brailowsky, & Will, (*Brain Repair*, 1995), our emotional and motivational states play a large role in how much and how fast we recover. Some motivated people even acquire new skills many years post-injury! *I learned to board- and kayak-surf 25 years later.*

Brain repair is remarkable and simple: this dynamic organ started with 100 billion *neurons* and even more interconnection, and can reorganize and reprogram itself. This occurs because of *neuroplasticity* — the brain's *neurons* can be remolded. The cells find new and better patterns. According to Stephen Stahl (*Essential Psychopharmacology*, 2000) and others, the *neurons* form new connections and remove old ones, branching and pruning — think of how a tree's branches change as the tree grows.

Recent research shows that new neurons do grow to replace the ones that died. Unfortunately the process takes a long time, but it may help to explain why people can keep on improving even years after their injury — and why maintaining a healthy lifestyle that leads to maximum growth is important.

How does *neuroplasticity* work?

Basically, the brain uses three processes to repair itself: *collateral sprouting, unmasking,* and *substitution of function.*

> Do not let what you cannot do interfere with what you can do.
> — Coach John Wooden

Collateral sprouting occurs when undamaged cells grow into an injured area after some or all of it has been destroyed. In this process, undamaged *neurons* sprout additional branches, which then extend into the spaces that were formerly occupied by the damaged or dead *neurons*. These new sprouts may be either from the same system or from another region.

Unmasking occurs when intact but previously unused or lesser *neurons* take over the role of the dead or damaged cells.

Then, in a molding process called *substitution of function*, the new *unmasked* neurons function to replace the injured brain cells. *Compensation* also occurs: a different set of healthy cells in another area can take over the role of those damaged.

After these *neuroplastic* changes, how will the brain work?
The new brain will likely work slower, but it will work. Without suggesting that the brain is "hard-wired," my favorite example explains the "rewiring": Imagine placing a telephone call between New York and Denver during a storm. Before the storm (pre-injury), a direct line was used. After the storm (post-injury), the direct lines are down, and an indirect route must be used — the call now must go through Chicago on its way to Denver. Thus, different/new lines are *unmasked*. While neither the quickness nor quality of the new after-storm connection is the same as the direct line, the call, nonetheless, does get through to Denver.

The phone lines respond like the "new" brain: with sufficient repetition, remaining fibers are strengthened and high efficiency can again be reached. The brain can adapt and compensate. And, although

> My pleasure lies in seeing that I myself grow better day by day.
> — Epictetus

the call still looks the same to the receiver, it doesn't act the same and it is more difficult to complete. But it's still a call. Just as some brain-injury survivors look the same, still work, and are still people — but may not act the same.

What can rehabilitation ("rehab") do for me? How does it help?
Rehabilitation can repair the break in the chain at its broken point — to start the rewiring process. The goals of rehabilitation are to:
- Make new connections.
- Join the newly repaired wires to the unbroken wires.
- Develop new performance goals.

Rehabilitation can help you relearn or adapt your skills. Because brain injury affects us in many different ways, our deficits are as varied as the functions of the brain. Thus, rehabilitation addresses several areas:
- Physical
- Cognitive
- Communication
- Psychological
- Behavioral
- Social

- Family
- Community
- Vocational

Does that list look overwhelming? Rehabilitation is a lot of work — but you want to get better, don't you? Not surprisingly, research has shown a strong relationship between effort and improve-

> Luck is a matter of preparation meeting opportunity.
> — Oprah Winfrey

ment. Although spontaneous recovery in the early weeks and months results in rapid progress, this is probably due to natural healing and return of function in structurally intact cells. Beyond that you need to persevere in a relearning and retraining process, during which you improve by repetition and adaptation — both internally (in your brain) and externally (in your world).

Rehabilitation can help you to learn "to do what you can with what you have," "to make the best of it," and "to make lemonade out of lemons." You learn to use what you have left and train your remaining cells to take over functions they weren't responsible for before the injury.

Good news! Even those who have not received intervention for several years — even up to 15 years! — may regain lost skills when therapy is begun again (Bray

> If you will it, it is no dream.
> — Theodore Herzl

et al., 1987). This is likely because of *neuroplasticity* — present in all but the very old — and because we learn new ways to compensate. Many factors affect recovery. A lot depends on your motivation.

Before beginning a mission, we need to take an inventory: What do we have? What do we need? Where are we going? What do we seek?

What do I need to do to recover and feel better?
Remember the messages in the *Rocky* movies:
- **Believe in yourself** — even just a little — to improve.
- **Work at getting better.** Like other physical organs, the more the brain is exercised and stimulated, the more efficiently it uses its resources. "Use it or lose it!"

- **Never ever quit.**
- **Establish short and long-term goals.** Write them down. Seeing where you've been can motivate you to keep reaching.

> Start by doing what's necessary, then what's possible, and suddenly you are doing the impossible.
> — St. Francis of Assisi

- **Learn what you can and cannot change**. Trying for years, without success, to "make it like it was" won't change what "is."
- **Ponder the Serenity Prayer**:

> God grant me the serenity to accept the things I cannot change, the courage to change the things I can, and the wisdom to know the difference
> — Reinhold Niebuhr

What traits do I need if I'm going to improve?

Perseverance is the most important trait. It means not quitting, even in the face of difficulties or lack of support by others. Others include:

- Motivation
- Goal-orientation
- Optimism
- Independence

> Perseverance is not a long race; it is many short races one after another.
> — Walter Elliott

An ability to recognize errors and an awareness of problem behaviors with enough mental flexibility to change — no different than from non-disabled people! — also plays a role in how much you recover.

How can I work on recovery at home and in my community?

Surround yourself with music that synchronizes your brain cells (see Chapter 4 "Spiritual Rewiring") and connect with people and things that enrich your life. *This doesn't mean connecting to the television!*

> The difference between achievers and non-achievers is a #2 pencil and a dream.
> — Jaime Escalante

Laboratory research demonstrates that rodents allowed to play with toys develop more connections between *neurons* than rodents raised in empty cages. The same is likely true for humans — even without cages!

And people who remain mentally active throughout life by reading, attending art events, and/or traveling keep their level of mental functioning longer — even compared to sedentary 20 year olds!

How do sensory-rich settings stimulate our brain cells? *Neurons* respond to stimulation by branching out and contacting more *neurons*, thus improving our functioning. The more we can activate our brain cells, the more we'll improve — it's that simple!

Research has found that the difference between those who continue to improve and others who stay the same or regress is that improvers stay busy. This busyness is usually a combination of many activities:

> If you're not growing, you're dying.
> — Anonymous

- Work of any variety, paid or unpaid.
- Study and educational experience: seminar, class, program.
- Hobbies, activities, games, sports.
- Social gatherings and community activities.
- Alone time — downtime away from overstimulation by people and places is a choice different from isolation and loneliness.
- A balance of activity and rest.

Can I rewire a paralyzed leg/arm/side? How?

Yes — if it is involved in activity and not neglected. Remember the phrase "use it or lose it"? One-sided neglect is most common after acute-onset brain injury such as *stroke* (brain damage from a

> Happiness walks on busy feet.
> — Kittie Turmell

hemorrhage or blockage of blood vessels), and frequently associated with *focal brain damage* (damage in a specific part of the brain), but it can occur with brain injuries of all types. The sure way to never regain any function is to act as though the limb is not there! As the following story shows, it is possible to improve if you work at it. By involving his injured side, this survivor was able to create some *collateral sprouting* and *unmasking* of the undamaged neurons, and thus, *substitution of function* occurred.

Internship, 1988

Ever the student of health and fitness, about 12 years after my brain injury I began a Master's degree program at San Diego State University on a part-time basis. To fulfill a requirement for practical experience to teach adapted Physical Education (PE), I chose to intern in a local community college's Adapted Aquatics Program.

> All things are possible until they are proved impossible — and even the impossible may only be so, as of now.
> — Pearl S. Buck

One of my assigned clients was a large man who weighed about 275 pounds and had recently sustained a brain injury from a stroke. "John" had one-sided neglect of his right arm and leg. The instructor, bless her soul, allowed me to trust my instincts regarding teaching methods as long as we achieved his goals.

After reading about various treatments for hemiparesis (paralysis of one side of the body), I was intrigued with the success of a method that involved talking to the injured part and acting "as if" it could function, so I tried it with "John." Talking to his injured side, I asked it to complete fewer of the same exercises than his uninjured side, and I encouraged "John" to continue the dialogue at home.

At the beginning, even I was somewhat skeptical that this would work. But, for lack of anything better, I continued talking, teasing, acting "as if." "John," too, was reluctant, but I convinced him to talk to his "bad side" — which we named "Ralph" so it wouldn't feel picked on!

Our goal, of course, was to get the injured side to work — and not just "go along for the ride." You can guess the rest: "John" gained some movement, and thus he increased strength and flexibility in his injured arm and leg — and reached his goals by the end of the semester!

Note: A research study demonstrated a 5% increase in muscular force when "you can do it!" was intoned during exercise! (Self, 1997)

Is there hope for me to recover — even after a severe injury?

Yes — if you work at it! *"It is not the kind of injury that matters, but the kind of head,"* says Sir Charles Symonds, a British neurologist. Every injury is different because every head (brain) is different. To use a computer analogy, the boxes may look the same, but it's what inside that matters!

Recovery depends on many factors, including your personality, lifestyle, work ethic, general health (e.g., smoking, substance use), fitness level (exercise), location/extent of the damage, social support system, kind/amount of rehabilitation, divine intervention, and luck!

If you sense — or heard, as I did — that doctors don't seem hopeful, remember that they don't know you. They can read a chart — but they cannot read determination. They can test for ability — but they cannot test for willingness to use

> Success isn't a result of spontaneous combustion. You must set yourself on fire.
> — Arnold H. Glasow

that ability. They can test for mental quickness — but not for mental courage. Only you and your family know the depth of your internal resources. The kind of brain that needs to rewire is the most critical factor for recovery. You can do it!

Summary

> When you can't solve the problem, manage it.
> — Rev. Robert H. Schuller

- Believe in yourself.
- You still possess a few billion *neurons* ready to work.
- Work at getting better.
- Strengthen some abilities, compensate for others, and adapt the environment.
- Find out what is and is not possible to change.
- Establish short and long-term goals.
- Some improvement can occur even years after an injury.
- "Use it or lose it!" and never ever quit.

4

Spiritual Rewiring: Healing Our Hearts with Prayer and the Arts

Bring yourself back to your heart center! Your soul and essence don't die in a brain injury.
— Chad Edwards, Founder, the Institute for Creative Living

This chapter explores practices to help you heal spiritually. By using music, other arts, and prayer, you can learn what can resonate within your soul to recreate yourself. The topics include:

- The "Mozart Effect": what music can do for me.
- How to chart your heart.
- Suggested music (composers and tunes) to suit your various moods.
- What is prayer? What prayers do people use?
- Health benefits of prayer — what can prayer do for me?
- If I'm not religious, then what?
- Ancient and current healing rituals and practices.
- Historical connection to the arts.
- How do healing rituals work? Why do I need them?
- How can I heal myself with art?
- Other expressive arts: visual, auditory, and physical arts.
- Receptive arts: listening, reading, watching, and enjoying arts.

Introduction

"Okay, prayer and the arts, like God and Mozart, right? How can they help? I don't need religion and culture now, thank you very much. Besides, this is a medical problem, so I'm looking for a medical solution. I'm not sure where to search, but I will continue my quest."

You've probably been on your quest for a while now. See if this describes you, even a little bit:

So far neither Western nor Eastern medicine "cures" have worked for me. As a good patient, I've endured EKGs, ENGs, ECTs, CATs, X-rays, and MRIs. I've been poked and probed, needled and noodled, pushed and pulled. I no longer even count the vials for all the blood tests!

And I've tried both mainstream and alternative therapies. But I'm not healed — I'm not whole even though tests show that my rewiring is finished, that my parts are rejoined, and that my body is fixed and no longer broken.

I feel everything but unified! I may look whole, healed, and connected. But I don't feel plugged in to myself — or anything else.

Maybe your parts have regained some old abilities and former speeds, but everything else in the world has upgraded skills and increased velocity! Can an antique car with new wires travel at current freeway speeds? Hardly. But is it happy to be restored? Maybe.

Your problem may not be having the speed to drive on the freeway or being linked with the mainstream. It may be you're not linked — period! And you fear that you never will be. You feel disconnected from yourself — who you are, who you were, and who you want to be. You need to heal your soul.

To feel whole again, you need to get to know your innermost self again! To find your soul and renew your spirit, you need to recover it. You need to find your heart center! How do you begin?

> When you have a disease, do not try to cure it. Find your center, and you will be healed.
> — Taoist proverb

Chart your heart!

How to Chart Your Heart

- **Why:** to discover a healthy sonic environment for your heart center.
- **What:** to find and explore your soul's sound preferences.
- **When:** at several times during your awake hours — perhaps at rising, late morning, afternoon, and evening — to respond to your variable stress levels.
- **Where:** a quiet space.
- **Equipment:** CDs and an appropriate player, iPod, or radio, notebook, pen, or pencil. If you need music ideas, see "Exploring Musical Selections to Create Moods."
- **Method:** listen to various kinds of music and observe how your body reacts. Then, record your responses to the following energy states using a scale from 1 to 10 or pluses (+) and minuses (-):

Physically Energizing .... Tiring
Pleasing.. Annoying
Cheering.. Depressing
Calming... Angering/Irritating

Here's a step-by-step plan:
- Block out other sights and sounds. Feel your heartbeat and pay attention to its rhythm.

> Music is the shorthand of emotion.
> — Leo Tolstoy

- Listen to your favorite kind of music/sounds/musician.
- Observe how your heart rate and mood respond.
- Record your responses to the energy states above, using a scale of 1-10 or pluses (+) and minuses (-).
- Change the musical selection — the track, artist or genre.
- Notice how your body responds to the different sounds.
- Repeat the steps.

Then choose and record the best music to help with these activities:
- Awakening.
- Eating.
- Physical tasks.

- Mental tasks.
- Socializing/conversing.
- Preparing to sleep.

For all activities, it is important to:
- Explore what kinds of noises short-circuit your brain and overwhelm you, requiring you to cover your ears and shut out everything. and
- Decide if neutral sounds (e.g., white noise made by an electric fan) help, hurt, or have no effect.

Now, apply what you learned about yourself to your daily activities. Listen to the music that resonates for each activity and — voila! — life is better for you and for everyone else!

What about noises that disturb me? What can I do?

To avoid distress and disharmony, first learn what sounds and noises overload your wires, then flee, fight, or negotiate. Here's how:

> By paying close attention to the pulse, pace, and pattern of music, you can create a sonic diet to keep you energized, refreshed, and relaxed throughout the changing seasons and cycles of your life.
> — Don Campbell

- **Flee.** Don't go there! Avoid them!
- **Fight back.** Use your own masking sounds or earplugs — or learn to meditate, so the sounds don't disturb you.
- **Negotiate.** Explain to the sound-maker why you need the noise reduced or stopped.

What happens when I chart my heart? How does it help me rewire?

When you chart your heart, when you respond to its beat, you begin to know how to heal your soul. You see how harmony heals and dissonance distresses, then you can rewire yourself to work at the correct speed to balance your "engine" — your heart center.

You and your heart center "car" may cough and sputter, stop and start. It'll probably be slow — occasionally you may get up to freeway speed. But don't count on daily trips on the superhighway, because you're not wired for that. You're wired for the scenic route. You've got a choice: stall on the freeway or meander on the back roads.

Respond to your heart center to heal your soul. Who knows what scenery awaits you? Maybe even peace and wholeness. Try it! A detour isn't a dead end unless you stop.

Think of this like making music. First, your internal conductors feel the rhythm. Then they give clear directions to your orchestra players so that they contribute their best efforts. When the movements of your inner symphony connect, you can act as a unified person — someone who is together. It can happen!

"Okay, fine," you say. "I'll listen, but I need help with the action. I'm brain-damaged, remember? I'll conduct this orchestra, but I'm new at this and don't know how to play all the instruments."

Not a problem. Healing with sound calls for both leaders and followers. Everyone plays a role in the recovery process. You don't need to do it alone. All you need to do is be receptive — to new ideas, to others, to the healing powers — and to try what feels right. You can heal your heart with prayer and the arts. You can play your own music. It's worked for years — many years. Now let's see how music can heal you.

Music

Before humans talked, we communicated primarily with sound or tone. Since ancient times, sound and music have been used to heal and protect. Music can calm your body, mind, and spirit to diminish pain, maximize intelligence, reduce anxiety, and increase coordination and productivity — with no side effects.

The Mozart Effect

Do you ever hum along with a tune in your head or on the radio? Does your mood reflect it? Can you sometimes not rid your mind of the song? Can you feel how your heart seems to match the pace of the music that you hear? Do your fingers begin to strum to the beat? These responses reflect the Mozart Effect: your brain waves and breathing patterns reflect the rhythms you hear.

Considered one of the world's most gifted classical composers, Wolfgang Amadeus Mozart composed music before he was five years old and worked feverishly until his untimely death at the age of 34. His music is recognized for its distinctive and upbeat sound.

We survivors can especially benefit from Mozart's music. Why? Regardless of musical preference, his melodies calm body and mind better than that of any other composer, according to the author of *The Mozart Effect*. And we all know that rewiring minds and bodies need peace! When we are calm, our thinking is clear — we can better control our emotions, and thus our behavior. *Not a bad idea for brain-injury survivors!* Other challenges, such as communicating and knowing where we are in space, improve too because certain music relaxes our bodies and stimulates our minds (Campbell, 1998).

To be more in synch, we're not limited to Mozart, either. Music by the composers Bach, Handel, Vivaldi, and Pachelbel also enables us to achieve relaxed alertness and concentration. See suggestions later in this chapter.

What occurs in my body when I hear music? (Campbell, 1997)

- Music affects breathing, heartbeat, and digestion.
- Music affects blood pressure and body temperature.
- Music can regulate brain waves.
- Music and sound can regulate stress-related hormones.
- Music can increase endorphin levels and boost immune function.
- Music reduces muscle tension and improves body movement.
- Music changes our perception of time and space.
- Music masks unpleasant sounds and feelings.
- Music can boost productivity, strengthen memory, and maximize ability to learn.
- Music can increase endurance.
- Music enhances romantic feelings and receptivity to symbolism.
- Music provides a safe expression of feelings and generates a sense of well-being.

> When I hear music, I fear no danger. I am invulnerable. I see no foe. I am related to the earliest times, and to the latest.
> — Henry David Thoreau

Want more benefits? (Cowley, 1998; Campbell, 1997, 1998)

- **Anxiety:** Listening to 30 minutes of classical music or taking 10 mg of Valium resulted in the same beneficial responses for heart patients.
- **Pain:** Migraine sufferers who were trained to use music, imagery, and other relaxation techniques reduced the frequency, intensity, and duration of their headaches.
- **Intelligence:** After "music warmed up their brains," students who listened to 10 minutes of Mozart before taking a college aptitude test scored higher than those not exposed to the music.
- **Performance:** Students who listened to music before taking a college aptitude test scored higher on both portions of the test (fifty-one points higher on verbal and thirty-nine points on math).

> You will experience the best healing results when you open up to listen not just with your physical ears, but when you start to feel the vibration of the music with your whole body and spirit.
> — Deuter

- **Productivity:** Manuscript editors who listened to 90 minutes of light classical music improved accuracy by 21%.

Music for Various Moods

To heal ourselves with music, it is essential to know what it does. What kinds of effects do different sonic environments produce? As we reconnect and rewire, how can we protect our fragile sound channels? How do the different musical types influence body, mind, and spirit? How can we create specific effects? What works to optimize sensitive wires under construction?

The following categories are only general classifications — a variety of styles harmoniously coexist within each musical genre. Jazz is a good example of a genre that offers tempos from hot to cool to fit our varying needs and moods. As we become aware of the different mood-altering effects that each kind of music delivers, we can create the proper environment. Don Campbell (1997) and I suggest:

To feel grounded, peaceful, spiritually aware, and even transcend pain: Sacred music, like drumming, church hymns, spirituals, and gospel music. *I awaken my system with choral music sung by the St. Olaf College (my alma mater) Choir or other gentle religious music.*

To reduce stress, meditate, study: Gregorian chant. These low tonal sounds create a sense of peace, relax, and evoke a sense of space.

For relaxed alertness: New Age or ambient music is effective because it displays no dominant rhythm and suggests endless time and space.

To stimulate the mind, improve concentration and memory: Classical music with a light melody is clear, elegant, and employs a constant, moderately fast beat with high frequencies.

To relieve anxiety and aid focus: Baroque music that is stable and orderly with a slow beat (60 beats per minute) and low tones, such as Vivaldi. *I also like nature sounds, especially forest or ocean.*

To unlock creative impulses and stimulate imagination: Two types work especially well:
- Upbeat instrumental music, with a basic but unpredictable structure that liberates your mind to roam, such as Beethoven's Pastoral Symphony and Dvorak's New World Symphony.
- Impressionist music, e.g., Debussy and Ravel, with free-flowing sounds evoking dreamlike images, unlocks creative impulses. *The "Out of Africa" soundtrack and any nature soundtrack send me dreaming.*

To enhance sympathy, compassion, and love: Romantic music of Schubert, Schumann, and Liszt emphasizes expression and feeling. *I like vocals by James Taylor, k.d. lang, Natalie Merchant, Ray Charles' "Genius Loves Company," and many by Eric Clapton.*

To uplift, inspire, and release deep feelings: Slow jazz and blues, and other music from the African heritage, including Dixieland, calypso, and reggae, were created to unlock emotions and inspire a

> Music washes away from the soul the dust of everyday life.
> — Berthold Auerbach

sense of common humanity. Listening to slow blues magically lifts the blues! *My favorites include: Paul Simon's "Graceland," Bruce Springsteen's "The Rising," Dixie Chicks, Ray Charles, and Billie Holliday. Don Campbell likes "The Lady Sings the Blues" soundtrack.*

To stimulate the body: Dance or swing music, , especially salsa, rumba, merengue, and other forms of South American music, uses a lively rhythm to energize, as does the *Flashdance* soundtrack and Irish dance music like Riverdance. Samba can both energize and relax. *I especially like the 1988 Olympic theme song and many by Stevie Ray Vaughn.*

To create a sense of well-being: Both vocal and instrumental versions fulfill this need. Top-40, country-western, pop, light jazz, big band, and renaissance wind music all stir emotions and inspire movement. *I like, "Ultimate Divas," Judy Collins, John Denver, and Fleetwood Mac.*

To stimulate active movement or mask loud/annoying noise: Rock music, either classic or contemporary, works wonders to drown diesel engines. *I also like Paul Simon's "Graceland," Janis Joplin, and the Indigo Girls. Don Campbell likes Elvis Presley.*

To relieve anger: Any intense, energetic, driven music helps to release strong emotions. Also, fast jazz and some symphony pieces (such as Brahms' "Piano Concerto") fill this need. Heavy metal, rap, hip-hop, etc. — music that suggests inner turmoil and a need for release — may work for some people. *I play fast Neil Diamond or tunes by Bob Dylan while I clean — cleaning is another good antidote for anger!*

Important: Follow up with relaxing pieces to restore your inner harmony.

Personal experience. For all moods, when a selection doesn't work or disturbs me, I use my SAFER plan (Stop, Assess, Fix, Evaluate, Retry). Then I can focus on whatever it is that I'm doing rather than using part of my brain to block out an offending sound.

Here are more ideas from Don Campbell and me:

Mood	Music
To feel peaceful, grounded, spiritual.	"Enchanted," "Healing Praise Songs," "Amazing Grace."
To reduce stress, meditate, study.	Gregorian chants, water sounds.
For relaxed alertness.	Steven Halperin, Enya, Paul Winter, "Lifescape" series, Mozart.
To stimulate the mind, improve concentration and memory.	Mozart, Haydn, Native American flute, wind music.
To relieve anxiety and aid focus.	Bach, Handel, Pachelbel, drumming.
To unlock creativity.	John Coltrane, Miles Davis, Kenny G, James Galway, nature sounds.
To enhance sympathy and love.	Tchaikovsky, Chopin, Norah Jones.
To uplift, inspire, unlock emotions.	Ladysmith, Black Mambazo, Eric Clapton, Indigo Girls.
To stimulate the body.	Motown, classic rock, Van Halen.
To create a sense of well being.	The Beatles, Neil Diamond, oldies.
To stimulate active movement & mask loud noise.	Rolling Stones, Bonnie Raitt, Dixie Chicks, oldies.
To relieve anger.	Bruce Springsteen, Janis Joplin.

Special Workout Tunes

Moving — whether walking, exercising, or working out — is often easier and more fun when we step to the beat of music we favor. Music not only keeps boredom at bay, but it also provides the workout our hearts need for fitness. Here are some special tunes (Dembling, 1998):

To warm up and cool down (115-125 beats per minute):
"All I Wanna Do," Sheryl Crow; "Graceland," Paul Simon; "I've Got My Love to Keep Me Warm," Ella Fitzgerald and Louis Armstrong.

To work at a steady aerobic pace (125-240 beats per minute):
"Gone," Dwight Yoakam; "Little Red Corvette," Prince; "That Old Black Magic," Louis Prima and Keely Smith.

These '60s oldies are fast and also good for workouts:
"Sugar Shack," Jimmy Gilmer & the Fireballs; "He's So Fine," The Chiffons; "It's My Party," Lesley Gore; "Louie Louie," The Kingsmen; "Walk Like A Man," The Four Seasons; "My Boyfriend's Back," The Angels; "Whole Lot of Shakin' Going On," Jerry Lee Lewis; "Surfin' USA," and others by the Beach Boys; "Peggy Sue," and others by Buddy Holly.

Top 10 running songs — these can work for any repetitive activity:
Theme from "Chariots of Fire"; "Born to Run," Bruce Springsteen; "Eye of the Tiger," Survivor; "Start Me Up," Rolling Stones; "Running on Empty," Jackson Browne; "Born to Be Wild," Steppenwolf; "Gonna Fly Now," theme from *Rocky*, Bill Conti; "Runnin' Down a Dream," Tom Petty and the Heartbreakers; "Run Like Hell," Pink Floyd; "Should I Stay or Should I Go?" The Clash.

Music for Stressful Times

How can I prepare myself for unavoidable stressors?
- Plan outings for times when disturbing noises are less likely to occur, e.g., weekday mornings and evenings are quieter times for shopping than lunch hour, rush hour, or weekends.

> When words fail, music speaks.
> — Hans Christian Andersen

- Arm yourself with your own sounds: CD player, iPod, etc.

- Experiment with/use earplugs or headphones of various types.
- Learn how to meditate. First practice in peaceful settings.

Personal experience. To prevent my wires from shorting out from loud noises, my former therapist Christine referred me to an audiologist who works with survivors who experience hyperacusis (super sensitivity to sound). By creating custom-made earplugs for me, the audiologist also validated that loud noises distressed me, which aided my self-esteem.

How can music help me with noise, stress, and overload?

Before your wires short, escape or fight back. Cover your ears and exit the painful place — fast! What if you can't escape — drown out the offending noise with your own soothing tunes, meditate, or ask the sound controller to reduce the volume, change the music, or turn it off. It's vital to not alienate those you ask for help — speak up before your wires are fried so your emotions won't control you!

Personal experience. When I lived in Leucadia, north of San Diego, my brain was continuously bombarded with train noise — either the lumbering freights or blasts of the commuter-train horns 100 yards away from my mobile home. At the first sound, I plugged my ears and ran as far away as possible. If I was on the computer, I plugged my ears and increased the volume of my music or quickly put on my headphones.

What do I do if my wires short?

Blown circuits call for two steps. First, if possible, play some soothing music on any available sound system or grab your headphones. If this is not an option, proceed immediately to grounding:

To ground yourself to the earth: from a seated position, place both feet flat on the floor or place your entire body on the floor, with either knees bent or flat. Breathe deeply. Closing your eyes can help. Stay there for as long it takes to feel calm again. After you feel rooted to the earth, give yourself permission to slowly resume activities. Associate only with peaceful people and treat yourself as you would an injured friend.

Personal experience. People we don't know may not understand our actions or the extent of the damage possible if we don't act. It probably doesn't matter if they're confused, if what we do can prevent an outburst. Friends will assist us if they know what to do.

Healing with Prayer

In what other ways can you respond to your heart center?
"When your mind is quiet, you lose your sense of separateness and isolation. You may even experience your higher self," according to Dean Ornish, MD, a well-known advocate of lifestyle practices like meditation and yoga (Cowley, 1998).

"What? This sounds like prayer! I need more than prayer now."

Wait a minute. Before you discard seeking your higher self as yet another crazy idea that won't work with a medical problem, hear me out:

> Let go and let God.
> — Anonymous

Isn't listening to the voice of our hearts like listening to God or whatever "higher power" we choose? Isn't God (or Goddess) within us, anyway? When we pray, we address not only the Ultimate, but also ourselves. When we speak or express in another way, we're talking to God. When we're silent or receptive, we're listening to God.

What Is Prayer?

"We shall overcome." "Go, team, go!" People pray all the time, although maybe not in the way that we normally associate with the word. Any repeated phrase can be considered prayer.

The word "prayer" simply means a plea or request directed at someone or something that we see as a power greater than ourselves. Sometimes the prayer request may feel like that still, small voice that yearns to be heard — like we feel much of the time. If we pray in a group setting, we may feel more powerful.

The answer? It may take a long time to come. We may not recognize it. It may knock softly. Or it can hammer on several levels. Some of us won't hear it unless it's a deafening slam similar to that from a two-by-four piece of wood. Our "higher power" will do whatever it takes to make us hear. All we need to do is listen — and then act. Action is essential!

A story about a man who didn't pay attention to God's answer:
During a raging flood, a man became stranded on the roof of his house. Rescuers in a rowboat came by and tried to coax him into the boat. "No!" he cried. "God is going to rescue me!"

While he continued praying, another rowboat came by, and again he refused to get in. "God is going to save me!" he said.

Then a helicopter flew over and tried to lower a rope ladder. The man waved it away. "God will rescue me. Go away!"

Finally the floodwaters rose and the man died. At heaven's door he bitterly demanded, "God! Why didn't You save me?"

> Call on God, but row away from the rocks!
> — Robert M. Young

"You idiot!" God replied. "I sent you two rowboats and a helicopter!"

What prayers do people use?
Buddhism: Believers may use a mantra — often intoning the centering "om" sound. The most famous mantra, "Om mane padme hum," meaning "All hail the Jewel in the Lotus," is designed to cleanse the six realms of all negative karmas from mind, body, and speech (Dharma Haven). Believers are urged to repeat this mantra 108 times while visualizing the light that emanates from the syllable "om" (Craughwell, 1998).

Christianity: For centering and guidance, followers say "The Lord's Prayer" and various psalms, proverbs, and songs from the Bible and other sacred readings, such as "The Twenty-third Psalm." Roman Catholics pray "The Hail Mary."

Personal experience. *To remind me to be my best self, I post copies of "The Prayer of St. Francis of Assisi" in several places. Even then, that other self still erupts. But what would happen if no prayers were posted!*

Lord, make me an instrument of your peace,
Where there is hatred, let me sow love;
where there is injury, pardon;
where there is doubt, faith;
where there is despair, hope;
where there is darkness, light;
where there is sadness, joy;

O Divine Master, grant that I may not so much seek to be consoled as
    to console;
to be understood as to understand;
to be loved as to love.

For it is in giving that we receive;
it is in pardoning that we are pardoned;
and it is in dying that we are born to eternal life.

Hinduism: Sacred texts, such as the Atharveda, contain magical healing "charms" that enable Hindus to achieve the sacred state of physical, mental, spiritual, and material wealth (Craughwell, 1998).

Islam: Muslims find solace in readings from their sacred book, the Koran, believed to be a revelation by God to the prophet and messenger Mohammed. The essential "Call to Prayer," said five times a day by the faithful, acts like a mantra (Craughwell, 1998).

Judaism: Followers obey what is written in the Torah. The Jewish tradition also includes study of other sacred texts such as the Talmud, the use of symbols, and daily prayer. One favorite prayer is "Hear O Israel."

> Where is God?
> God is where we let Him in.
> — Rabbi David Frank

I'm new at this prayer thing. How do I pray?
The best place to start is from own your faith tradition. If this is new to you, investigate the spirituality section of any good bookstore or visit

places of worship to find what resonates. Whatever feels good for your heart center is what will heal your soul — no matter what it's called. Every spiritual tradition uses several different ways to connect to the Divine.

Well-known Christian leader Norman Vincent Peale advised: to start by finding a quiet space to be alone:

> In every culture, there's a belief in powers, forces, energy out there. It's as if we're wired for God, as a survival instinct. Believing in the Almighty… gives us strength and solace … healing in the truest sense of the word.
> — Herbert Benson, MD

- Relax the body, empty the mind of all problems, and focus the spirit on God.
- Talk simply — about anything.
- Speak in your normal mode.
- Ask for what you want.
- Accept whatever God delivers.
- Pray for strength to do your best, then confidently leave the rest to God.
- Pray frequently, wherever you are. Shut out the world and talk to God to remind yourself of the nearness of the Divine.

The secrets to prayer are simplicity, practice, faith, and acceptance — all delivered with positive thoughts. Believe that you will be answered and then "let go and let God."

Prayer aids are used by worshippers in all religions to help focus attention, achieve the desired peaceful state, and provide a further connection to the Divine, particularly if the item is blessed by a church official or shaman. Prayer aids include pictures, beads, shawls, rocks, amulets, incense, candles, Tibetan singing bowls, icons, totems and written verse — anything that fosters a bond.

The comfortable routine of a familiar item and the repetitive motions that are used, e.g., beads or totems, help to create peace and balance that aids focus. Incense is often thought to enhance a meditative state, both by its historical connection to mysticism and the powers of its perfumes.

What can prayer do for me? What are the health benefits?
How about relaxing, reducing stress, and generally improving mood? Prayer can remind us of our connections — to Creation, others, and self — and that we are not alone in a crazy universe. Asking for help and voicing our fears also takes them outside of ourselves, thus they become easier to handle.

Improved health is documented in 212 studies that examined the effects of religious commitment on such outcomes as reduced blood pressure, depression, and anxiety; 75% demonstrated the value of faith. And, significant health benefits built up, even if prayer recipients were strangers! (Williams, 1996).

We don't know whether the better health shown in this research was due to other factors, such as group support or even that religious people follow more health practices in general. But we do know that all went to their place of worship and prayed. Try this for yourself and see!

> A soul should always stand ajar, ready to welcome the ecstatic experience.
> — Emily Dickinson

So, is prayer like a divine credit card? What won't prayer do?
Not exactly. It's more mysterious than "buy now, pay later" because we're not in control of whether a prayer will be answered — if, when, or how. As in any relationship, the outcome is not certain though we can be open to receive whatever comes. Hopefully we can remember to "let go and let God," although some of us like to hang on. Maybe we can ask for freedom from this need to cling?!

Prayer won't always give us what we want, or how, or when. This is the scary part — it's not like a credit card — we don't get to choose what comes our way. Our prayers may not even be answered in a way we understand right now. Perhaps the answer comes in the form of a

> Our rabbi once said, "God always answers our prayers; it's just that sometimes the answer is no."
> — Barbara Feinstein

question or another challenge or in the person of a stranger — remember the story about the man in the flood who waited for God's help.

Personal experience. Earlier I mentioned my epiphany in the late
'70s about the reason for all my pain. Here's a recap: as I returned from
my weekly visit to my shrink, the traffic light on my off-ramp turned red,
and my journey — and inner dialogue — suddenly halted.

"Now *I know why I'm getting all this s---! It's because I'm stronger
than many others, so I must carry their burden as well as my own! Oh
great,"* I thought, *"Well, what if I don't* want *to carry such a big load?"*

"*I'm sorry, my dear child,"* spoke a far-off voice. *"You don't choose
the size of the burden. I do — and I selected you for this because you're
so special."*

"*Wow! I'm chosen — what a difference* that *makes! Rather than
punished for being weak, I'm chosen because I'm strong! Okay, let the
games begin anew! — I finally get it! I don't like it, but I understand now.
If that's what God wants — then who am I to question such an
outrageous idea? I've always rather liked outrage, anyway, haven't I?"*

If I don't feel a direct connection to God, how do I pray?
Spirituality is about exploring inner lives,
however creative that may be. Prayer can
be directed wherever we choose.
Whatever we see as the ideal or highest
power in our lives — that Something
larger than ourselves — receives our healing requests. Through the ages,
in different faith traditions, people have sought intermediaries to God.
Depending upon cultural and religious experiences, various ones are
chosen. See *Brain Injury Rewiring for Loved Ones* for further discussion.

> There are many paths
> up the mountain.
> — Rabbi Marc Gellman

What kinds of healing rituals and practices do people use today?
Today's healing rituals integrate worldwide cultural practices. More than
just providing comfort, rituals are balms for what ails us — whether we
recite a prayer, intone a word, focus on a specific image, or perform a
physical motion. Many survivors gain comfort from rituals.

African Spirituality: Dancing and drumming are vital to many healing
traditions. These repetitive rhythmic movements induce an ecstatic state

that first stimulates and then relaxes the mind and body with the change in focus from the self to the activity (Hirsch, 1993).

Buddhism: To believers, meditation is the way to Enlightenment, which is the discovery of one's own true nature. To help achieve a state of non-attachment during meditation, practitioners perform three main activities to simultaneously occupy mind, speech, and body: mantra recitation, visualization of the Buddha, and special postures and gestures called "mudra" (Dharma Haven).

Christianity: Christians follow the example of their most famous healer, Jesus Christ, using the laying on of hands. To soothe and calm and to pass the love and energy from the healer to the recipient, hands are typically placed on both shoulders. A priest or other healer anoints the forehead of ill parishioners with oil. Healing prayer may involve ministers, the use of oil, the laying-on of hands to ask God to heal specific symptoms — directing all energies toward the same goal. If imagining "healing" is too abstract, picture "good guys" gobbling up "bad guys."

Prayer lists of people with special needs may be read at weekly services, prayed for by groups, or posted in the church bulletin.

Prayer chains are traditional in the Christian community. Connected by telephone or email, church volunteers pray for people whose names are offered by themselves or others.

Personal experience. With my frequent injuries, I was a regular participant at special healings with oil that were offered bi-weekly and at special occasions following communion at St. Michael's Episcopal Church in Carlsbad, CA. Whenever I received communion while wearing a brace or bandage, priests also added a healing. I always felt a sense of warmth and a reduction in pain, if not a faint electric current. Currently, I experience the same benefits from the prayer teams after communion at St. Paul's Episcopal in Ventura, CA.

Hinduism: Regular fasting is practiced by many who believe that it cleanses the body of impurities. Devotees also fast on behalf of a relative in the hope of pleasing a god who can bestow health (Cool, 1997).

Islam: Special verses from the Koran are read to Muslims who are ill to encourage patience and aid compliance with the tenets of Islam, which means submission to the will of Allah (Cool, 1997).

Judaism: Important practices include prayer and fasting to atone for sins on Yom Kippur, the most important religious holiday. Orthodox Jews rock in a heel-to-toe fashion as an aid to worship. In keeping with the communal nature of the religion, temple members visit people who are sick (Epstein, 1998).

Native American: To attain a meditative state of prayer and purification as an aid to healing, the traditional sweat lodge ceremony is still practiced by numerous Native American tribes today. Acting on the belief that sweating rids the body of illness and heals the spirit, participants gather in a sweat lodge to inhale steam from hot rocks, sing, and pray either with or on behalf of an ill member (Barfield, 1998).

Sand painting is used by several tribes, created by a medicine man who recounts a traditional healing story to a patient placed on the ground and encircled by members of his tribe. The shapes and colors are believed to reach the spirits and heal the patient.

Syncretism: This merges Native American spirituality practices such as the sweat lodge ceremony and Catholic traditions such as the Mass.

What are some other important healing practices?
Tai Chi: These moving meditations that mimic shadow boxing provide a spiritual workout for practitioners of many persuasions, particularly followers of Eastern religions. Deliberate breathing and ritual movement help focus the mind.

Yoga: This set of physical and mental exercises is often performed to chanting or other music to produce spiritual enlightenment. Hindus and worshippers of other faiths practice this regimen. Yoga practice starts with the mutual greeting of "namaste," which means "the Divine in me honors the Divine in you." To attain the necessary focus, mindful breathing and tonal sounds such as "om" often follow and precede the practice of postures. See Chapter 10 "Physical Rewiring" for more information.

Meditation: This state of mindful focus practiced in diverse religious and philosophic traditions may be identified by different names and varying forms, but all seek the same goal — an inner peace and calm that leads to balance.

Regardless of religious belief — or no religious belief at all — this technique is practiced throughout the world — and has been for ages. Typically, people who meditate silently repeat a word or phrase, called a mantra, for 20-minute sessions once or twice a day. When an outside thought intrudes, first it is acknowledged, then meditators turn their attention back to the mantra. No self-criticism or value is placed on the intruding thought — just acceptance, which leads to a calm state. Many people who meditate choose a prayer as their mantra (Williams, 1996).

How can I learn to meditate? I'm brain-damaged.

Survivors are good candidates for meditation because we tend to zone out a lot! To be effective, do it purposefully — just like prayer. At first, meditate at a special time and in a quiet place, rather

> Some things have to be believed to be seen.
> — Ralph Hodgson

than haphazardly or in response to sensory overload. Meditation need not be passive. Moving mediations, like tai chi, may work better for active or restless people. Any phrase that works to create a sense of peace is a meditation. *I often use a mantra to run faster and to calm me, saying, "Fast and light."*

Many options are available for learning meditation because research studies now demonstrate the strong connection between stress and health problems. Ask one of your medical professionals, and check with your local hospital, community health services, or adult education center about local resources for learning yoga.

The Arts

Art is as old as people. Historians date the first healing rituals to the hunter-gatherer cultures. Worldwide, for tens of thousands of years, wherever human beings lived, they called upon the healing power of music, dance, and other arts to connect people with their higher power, each other, and their inner spirit.

Traditional cultures believed that art healed the world as well as the individual. To connect — whether with God, a higher power, the universe, or Mother Earth — is a universal need. And all of humanity seeks a power outside itself to overcome earthly obstacles.

All of the arts are believed to have originated with the spiritual craft of shamanism in which gifted healers connected the higher consciousness and the ordinary — spirits and people. To bridge the worlds in their healing ceremonies, shamans used the tools of music, sound, and charms.

Through the medium of sound, believed to magically connect the powers above and below, the shamans called on the great spirits to heal individuals, families, and tribes. These rituals blended three elements: the shaman, the patient, and the invisible spirits that do the work between the worlds of heaven and earth. Involvement by each element was vital to the success of the cure, as were the family, community, and traditions.

The practitioner — priest or priestess — incorporated shared cultural myths, images, symbols, and objects into the ancient healing process. Music was used to assist the person with the disease to integrate mind and body in the recovery process — the current of sound quickened the healing of both physical and mental health.

What kinds of healing ceremonies did the ancients practice? Why?
Praying. Clapping. Drumming. Dancing. Toning. Chanting. Singing. Shouting. Practicing these activities maintained a connection to their higher power and to their ancestors. Connecting to the spirits through the arts, they sought healing at many levels: to improve health, wealth, and happiness; to instill a common vision; to affirm order; to perpetuate cultural values; to appease ancestors; to protect against evil influences such as demons of illness and bad luck; to discover hidden truths; to divine the future; and, ultimately, to achieve ecstasy.

Whether sonic healing comes from Tibetan singing bowls, Indian mantras, African drummers, or Celtic strummers, common goals, themes, and patterns emerge from this tradition. And whether invoking the spirits for crop success or birth, death, or marriage, these seasonal ceremonies promoted harmony and balance within the tribe, between men and women, and with the natural elements (Phoenix & Arabeth).

What happened during the ceremonies?

Directed by a shaman, members of a tribe danced wildly and then entered a trance or meditative state. It was believed that the dance freed the "boiling energy" — healing spirit could be freed from within each person with full participation in the art and music "space" of a ritual.

This ceremony eventually evolved into one that included costumes, storytelling, objects, and painting — this combination is called theater or performance art. However, in ancient times, the ritual was sacred and tied in with the culture's medicine. That sacred music, song, and dance were a gift of the gods was a belief shared by many cultures, so it was natural for medicine and the arts to merge to promote total healing (Grey).

Why do I need healing rituals? How do they work?

Why — because you can heal yourself and lift your spirits! Rituals use repetitive motion, chant, or prayer that not only provides comfort but also leads to relaxation — which in turn strengthens your immune system, so it can better fight off invaders and shore up resources to maintain health and balance.

Living is stressful, especially for your loved ones and you. Nothing is automatic anymore after your injury; you always need to "put in a work order" to your brain — your body responds to your demands by increasing pulse and blood pressure, speeding up your brain waves, and tensing your muscles. While this is a "fight or flight" response to stress, you only need it in emergencies. Sometimes your body acts like it's a normal state. To avoid stress-caused illness, you need to avoid this "on call" status of your system.

One researcher, Herbert Benson, MD, author of *Timeless Healing: The Power and Biology of Belief* (1996), estimates that 60% to 90% of all visits to doctors are the result of illnesses caused by mental stress (Cool, 1997).

How can prayer, meditation, music, or ritual reduce stress?

Repetitive activities create the relaxation response, a physiological state of slow, deep breathing and lowered heart rate. Natural to these activities that bring calm, peace, and harmony are several important elements including higher power and focus. *Sounds like my original themes of God, inner drive, and helpers, doesn't it?*

When people with chronic pain achieved the relaxation response, they reduced their visits to doctors by one-third and 75% of people who suffered from insomnia slept normally. According to Dr. Benson, "To the extent that a condition is caused or worsened by stress, relaxation techniques can cure or improve it." (Cool, 1997).

Personal experience. During especially stressful periods, I used to rock continuously, whether standing or sitting. For example, during my hearing to determine eligibility for Social Security benefits, before brain injury was considered a category, I needed to qualify as someone who was mentally ill. And so, as I rocked in my chair for 2½ hours, my wise attorney did not halt it. At the end of the hearing, the judge asked me if I realized that I'd rocked in my chair the entire time. My counsel said that I delivered a classic response: "Yes, your honor. I find myself rocking in church all the time, too." End of hearing. Benefits granted — this one is definitely mentally ill! Repetitive motion works on many levels!

Today, more than thirty years post injury, I still find myself rocking when my voice needs to be quiet but my body needs to move. Now, rather than feel mentally ill, I trust my body's wisdom as it rocks unconsciously until my mind is quieted by the repetitive activity.

Expressive Arts

In addition to music, prayer, and spiritual practices, various art forms can play vital roles to reconnect and heal all of us at the heart center. If we create harmony within, we may be able to demonstrate harmony without — first once, then occasionally, then more frequently!

"First you tell me prayer and Mozart can heal me. Fine. I try to meditate and listen to classical music when I read, eat, and rest. I will admit I feel more relaxed and centered in my mind, but my body is restless. I'm an active type of person and I need some action!"

> Use what talents you possess: the woods would be very silent if no birds sang there except those that sang best.
> — Henry Van Dyke

How can I actively heal myself with art?

If making music is not your artistic choice, select appropriate music to play. Then see yourself as an artist. Go ahead! Daydream!

Do you see yourself as an illustrator, painter, sculptor, or photographer? If you're playful, you may want to be an animator! Perhaps you see yourself as a musician. Maybe woodcarving fascinates you. Remember the models you used to build? Go back and rediscover the joy of creative activity — or start now!

As a survivor, you probably have many stories to tell, so writing may be a good choice, either poetry or prose. To capture these stories, either write or record them — maybe you can sell one or more!

Speaking of talking, maybe investigate radio. Ham or internet radio can be fun. Follow your heart. If your first choice loses its appeal, pick another one. Don't just think about it; do it! None of those "If I were…" excuses!

> Imagination is the true magic carpet.
> — Norman Vincent Peale

You are who you are now. Explore your interests and then act on them. You may discover hidden talents. Optimize your abilities. Make, do, create — something! You can always change it or discard it. And you don't have to journey the artistic path alone, unless that is your choice. All communities offer classes and groups of like-minded artists where, importantly, the focus is on the art — not on the disability!

I'm not an artist! What art can I possibly create?

Whatever you can imagine. You are an artist — you just need to discover your art; many forms await you. Keep an open mind and trust yourself.

Maybe free your powerful, inner healing spirit and stimulate your creative juices with Nature. Visit a park, forest, beach, or mountain and capture God's artistry on film, paper, or canvas. If you don't feel brave enough yet to create something, copy what you see at an art museum, in person, or on line, or investigate art books in a library. When we explore beyond our daily world, our horizons expand in other areas, too.

Rather than seek perfection and invite frustration and failure, seek to enjoy the act of creation. You only fail if you do nothing. Besides, you're new at this, so you get to make beginners' mistakes. And it's not just the product. It's the creative process — absorb yourself in what can be a fun and sometimes-messy adventure. Play some inspirational music. Part of the fun of rewiring is rediscovering what the new person loves to do.

Creating art is not only about what we make but also about what we do with what we make. Show it? Hide it? Destroy it? Your choice — your creations can be visible signs of your healing.

On those days when you don't feel creative, paint-by-number kits can keep you going. It's fun to make collages out of photos and advertisements in magazines. Maybe you and some friends can select a theme for your project. It's a relaxing way to rediscover what appeals to you and

> No great artist ever sees things as they really are. If he did, he would cease to be an artist.
> — Oscar Wilde

deepens relationships when you discuss your selections. Give yourselves a time limit such as one afternoon, so you can gain closure.

Personal experience. For me, enjoying an activity means finding one that suits both my limitations and abilities. If I struggle, it's not fun, I won't do it, and it doesn't help me. Nothing is gained except more stress — definitely not the goal here! So I assess my mood to see if I feel like investigating something new and possibly difficult or if I need the comfort of a safe, successful activity. The answer helps me decide what to do. Another option is to partner with a skilled friend and do it together!

Okay, I'll try to create art. But how can it heal me?
Art can transport you somewhere else, to a safe place. A sense of calm and peace can pervade you — almost a balanced feeling.

Just like music, other arts change us mentally, physically, and emotionally. We escape who we are and where we are. We're free of our earthly limitations. When we're relaxed, our physiology and attitudes change. You know the high you get when you exercise? We can experience a similar but different high when we venture into our own inner worlds — the world of our spirits and our souls.

Remember that, in general, healing occurs when our immune system operates optimally. When we control our inner state of serenity, our brains work better. When our brains work better, they heal us more efficiently — no longer awaiting the next fight or flight emergency.

Emotionally, art heals us beyond the creative process and the opportunity to escape from reality — without being medicated. It also provides that special sense of closure we get when we make something — even if we destroy it. Regardless of merit, the art we made is something of which we can be proud. And — if we feel brave enough — we can explore its meaning.

How often to create? Some of us need a daily artistic release; others only need to create weekly. To discover what works, try several different schedules, then write the current best one on a calendar. Scheduling

> Art is the only way to run away without leaving home.
> — Twyla Tharp

your creative time needs to reflect your changing needs — if last month's schedule no longer works, change it! Blocking "creative time" into your schedule may change bad days into good days!

Personal observation. *I remember making some clay pieces that I liked when I made them — and then later thought they were awful. So what? Making them was good at the time, which was all that mattered. I kept at it, improved, and then went on to something else, richer for the experience. "It was good when it was good" applies to many things!*

How can I, with my brain injury, create art?
Brain-damaged isn't brain-dead. Your soul didn't die, even if parts of your body did. A brain injury can actually help you to create art.

"What? This I gotta hear!"

Okay. First, for all of us, expressive arts make use of our natural inclination to return to the beginning. For better or worse, we recreate ourselves following injury. While we may often feel emotionally like children, also like them, we are free to express our heart centers openly. Brain injury makes natural and fearless creativity a reality again.

Second, older adults with life experiences return to this intrinsic mode of expression with another advantage — you know what works. You can trust your gut reactions because they are honed by your pre-injury experiences. *Finally — something that's better post-injury!*

Third, survivors tend to crave the comfort of sameness, of repetition. We like knowing what to expect. Art requires practice, just like any other skill. We do well what we do a lot. (How many of us forget how to eat?)

Fourth, survivors usually have plenty of time to explore and practice. Freeing the spirit, gathering materials, setting the environment, creating, cleaning up — all take time. Creativity cannot be rushed. This is good, because most of us don't like to be rushed, either.

If you're physically impaired, use what you've got. If one arm doesn't work, use the other one. If neither of them works, use your mouth, like some painters. Maybe talk into a tape recorder or use a computer voice recognition program if physically writing is too difficult.

Personal experience. *As a survivor-athlete, I am usually injured to some degree from some sports mishap. So, naturally during the long journey of writing* Brain Injury Rewiring, *it happens that I've been injured and/or ill a lot. Some of my conditions affected me mentally and emotionally but didn't impact the physical act of writing. Others directly affected the act of writing — but didn't stop it!*

I'll never forget the comment my kind therapist Christine made one time after I'd injured my thumb in a cycling accident. When I complained about the pain when I used the mouse on my computer, she said, "Use the other arm!" Rather than anger me, her comment propelled me to new thinking. I didn't seek an excuse — I sought an answer. Big difference!

Fortunately, due to multiple injuries, I am somewhat ambidextrous, so it was not impossible to use my other arm. It was slower, but like the rewiring of our brains, it still worked — just not as well. I also put on my scientific hat to analyze the problem: It turned out that my new "ergonomic" keyboard forced my arm into a stressful position. I immediately returned to using my smaller, older keyboard. Eureka! — no more pain! It's my SAFER (Stop, Assess, Fix, Evaluate, Retry) technique in action!

Visual Arts

Whether we paint with sand like ancient healers or sculpt with modern plastic materials, working with art media can satisfy the urge to express a variety of emotions for anyone, regardless of talent.

> A good snapshot stops a moment from running away.
> — Eudora Welty

Restoring emotional balance and a sense of meaning and order to life can result from simply freeing the mind to express itself. Consider: drawing by hand or on a computer, painting with acrylics or watercolors, sculpting with clay or plastic, sewing, knitting, or other needlecraft activities. Also consider:

Photography. Invest in an inexpensive digital camera. You can download pictures onto the computer, manipulate the images, then choose which ones to print. Numerous settings offer opportunities to experiment.

Filmmaking can be a fun way to get outside yourself, watch others, and create! Maybe borrow someone's video recorder or find a used one. Ask friends to join you for a fun social activity.

Puppets and masks can be constructed for use in theater or just for their art. Ancient healers used masks to embody specific spirits — think Halloween. When they wore the mask, they took its "spirit" onto themselves. It's also a good way to laugh, which we all need.

Auditory Arts

Singing or playing musical instruments, either alone or with others, provides not only a creative physical and emotional release but also raises intellectual abilities — so get musical and get smart (Campbell, 1997). Making music as a

> A bird does not sing because it has an answer. It sings because it has a song.
> — Chinese Proverb

member of a group also fosters a sense of belonging that survivors don't often experience.

What instrument can I play? I'm disabled and not musical.

Not musical? Says who? Community groups that provide a variety of musical opportunities at different skill levels await you. Investigate your local listings for adult education or recreation offerings and go! Just do it!

Let's start with your voice — the original healing instrument. In this return-to-the-beginning stage you are in, exploring the many sounds of this sonic tool can be a fun new activity. Remember to wear your non-judgmental hat! Accompanying performers from your favorite CDs might be a good way to start. Other ways to vocalize include:

Toning. Holding an elongated vowel sound for an extended period is a vocal activity that can be done anywhere, anytime, for free. By filling your body with oxygen, relaxing muscles, and stabilizing emotions, toning can release you from psychological and physical pain and relieve stress. An ancient method of healing, it is most often associated with Gregorian chants in which sounds like "om" are held. Humming is a quiet form of toning.

A toning program may start with five minutes of humming the first day. Follow this with the "ah" sound, which we all emit when we're relaxed. Then tone the most stimulating sound, "ee," which "awakens mind and body as a kind of sonic caffeine." Day four is reserved for the richest sound, "om." The next day can be one of exploring your vocal range, starting with the lowest vowel sound (Campbell, 1997).

Personal experience. After my injury, I could sing before I could talk. After discovering this phenomenon at a warm and accepting Methodist church at the University of Minnesota, I've sung in the choirs of whatever church I attended. Gratefully, I again sing with Master Chorale of Ventura County after a 2½-year absence because I failed two auditions. After pouting for two years, I joined another group, Gold Coast Concert Chorus, working very hard at home and at rehearsal. When the choirs combined for a concert, I practiced with both groups, finally performed well, and was invited to return!

Other instruments. Consider the harmonica — it's small, inexpensive, and easy to learn. If you're more inclined to use your hands, keyboards are fun. They also help to teach your ear to listen to music. If you've always wanted to play the guitar, try a "starter" guitar or ukulele, or maybe a dulcimer, which is three-stringed and easier to learn. Drumming provides the same benefits, whether you drum like the ancients or in an organized musical group, because of the way the body responds to the repetitive action. Other percussion instruments, e.g., cymbals, rattles, and bells, are inexpensive. Or find some in your kitchen!

If finances are a problem, check with your local music store about rent-to-buy programs and/or used instruments. Check out the want ads and pawnshops. Ask community college or adult education instructors.

And as the rhythm of Mozart's music unifies body and mind, so does the cadence of Shakespearean verse. The pattern of alternating spoken stresses called iambic pentameter matches the human heart rate of 65 to 75 beats a minute, just like the music of Mozart.

Talking aloud to yourself works — just watch your surroundings!

Personal experience. As a Sixties hippie wanna-be, I'd always envied guitar players, so I purchased a three-string dulcimer from a local music store, listened

> All art, like all love, is rooted in heartache.
> — Alfred Stieglitz

attentively, bought some books, and took it home. I promptly returned for instruction when I discovered my sound didn't mimic the sound of the storekeeper! It was fun to accompany myself as I sang choir songs and old favorites, especially during the cold, rainy, winter season.

Creative Writing

Relieving pent-up emotions through spoken or written voice is a cathartic healing experience — and available at any time! Writing poetry is a popular release for many people — especially when hurting — and crafting short stories or prose poetry is fun. Creating on the computer works for many of us because of organized files, easily altered material, and bypassing any physical weakness. If typing is too laborious, consider computer "voice-speak" programs. Adult education classes are available.

Journaling, a word used today to describe writing in a notebook, is another effective method of emotional release. The stream-of-consciousness technique, where thoughts are written without regard to spelling or grammar, is especially liberating. With a free flow of ideas, feelings of anger and hurt can be acknowledged and may be shared with someone who is not judgmental.

Because feelings often come in several layers, it will be necessary to spend more than one session uncovering them. One benefit of this technique is clearer self-understanding. Another is social — relating to others is easier when we are more together and balanced. Journaling also provides a record that can remind us how far we have come.

Personal experience. *As a poet since childhood, I used to feel sad when I read my published pre-injury verse. But I also read what I wrote when I was really crazy — and rejoiced that I'm not there now!*

Theater Arts

Acting can transport us somewhere else — and we get to be someone else! Don't escape through drugs. An invented story, costumes, make-up, and props can take you somewhere far better!

Improvisation games can be fun! Try shooting sounds to one another, dubbing voices (you gesture while another talks) or tell a story using another's hands. Other improv games can be found online.

Stagecraft offers another theater experience if you're not interested in acting. Local theaters always seek volunteers to build sets and make props.

Personal experience. *One winter I invited two of my friends to join me in an improvisational class that was offered at a local community college. On the first night I laughed more than in the previous month! Improv is the perfect theater for survivors because it's based on something we're very good at — impulsive behavior! There is no failure because there is no right way to do it.*

I need to be outdoors. What art can I do outside?
Besides photography, you can garden or build sandcastles or sand paint at the beach or in a box or in a lot at home. Maybe photograph your garden!

> *Personal experience. My brothers spent many hours every summer in the sand yard that was cleverly constructed beneath the kitchen window to give my parents a free babysitter. The boys were in the "army stage" then, building elaborate forts, complete with waterways, which they then took turns destroying — to build again another day.*

Gardening can also be a spiritual experience. And, whether plants flower abundantly or not, your soul will enjoy the weeding and tilling. See Chapter 10 "Physical Rewiring" for more information.

> *Personal experience. When I owned a mobile home, I raised roses because of their beauty and to honor my father who grew and gave away many beautiful blooms. My roses were his roses because I sprinkled some of my father's ashes on each new batch of compost.*
>
> *As I weeded my rose beds, I often weeded my life, too. As such, it was a continuous process as sometimes weeds masqueraded as desirable plants, only to disappoint me later. It also works the other way — what seem like weeds can have beautiful flowers.*

Physical Arts

You may not be able to talk or walk like you did pre-injury, but because "your soul doesn't die in a brain injury," you can still explore what brings you joy and integrate those activities into your life.

Remember our goal of regaining balance? At birth, our conductors (our brains) orchestrated our symphony to play in perfect harmony. All our organs played their parts to the beat of the heart and lungs, from neurons firing to food digesting. Then, our bodies worked as a harmonious whole. Now, after brain injury, they do not. Our rhythms no longer synchronize. To achieve balance and harmony, we need to recover that lost rhythm.

How can rhythmic activities help me create? I'm mobility-impaired.
Regardless of your level of mobility, something moves — allow it! Select some favorite tunes. Then, wearing your scientific (non-judgmental) hat, return to a childlike state and respond to different music, regardless of physical impairment. Explore how your body naturally moves to different rhythms and melodies. Watch it reflect joy, sadness, anger, peace. See how your pace changes. Let the music guide you to create various positions.

If you use a wheelchair, the wheels act as your legs as your arms direct the movement of the chair. You're only imprisoned by limitations you place on yourself. *Free your spirit and your body will follow.*

Dancing includes structured and practiced poses in ballet and modern dance as well as free dancing — move however you want! Any rhythmic movement lifts the spirits by raising

> Those move easiest who have learned to dance.
> — Alexander Pope

endorphin and serotonin levels. Classes and videos can provide instruction. Maybe invite friends to join you, wherever you dance!

Another way to respond to music is to play the role of a conductor of an orchestra. This can also be a good workout!

My creative-movement spirit is trapped! How can I let it out?
Go to a pre-school and watch the children. You'll return with a renewed sense of freedom. Start in a seated position and just move your arms in response to the music. Next, walk or roll your chair and move more body parts as you are led by your spirit! Gradually, you begin to dance!

> We can complain that the rose plant has thorns or rejoice that the thorn plant has roses.
> — Anonymous

Receptive Arts

Regardless of the ways you choose to receive the arts — whether you embrace the sights, sounds, and smells of nature; enjoy visual art in museums or galleries or written art in books; hear the artistic words and sounds created by various musicians and poets; or immerse yourself in cinema or theater arts — when you open your spirit and your self to the healing inherent in the arts, you heal on a deep level.

Personal experience. I find that I feel the most balanced and at peace when I attend a live performance, so I look for something every week. Fortunately, I usher at a nearby theater and local college performances are inexpensive, so this usually happens!

Summary

I hope that "Spiritual Rewiring" inspired you to create more than art — a new faith in prayer, yourself, and your abilities — as you heal yourself. I hope, too, that you discovered how the arts can reconnect you — at your heart center — with yourself and others. Expanded horizons — and friends — await you if you dare to explore this dynamic new path to harmony.

> Live a balanced life —
> learn some and think
> some and draw and
> paint and sing and
> dance and play and
> work every day some.
> — Robert Fulghum

You're the conductor on this trip as you chart your heart and journey to greater health and wellness. No one path will transport you all the way — but you must keep moving. You only fail if you stop.

- Chart your heart.
- Play the music that's best for each of your activities.
- Learn what sounds and noises overload your wires, then flee, fight, or negotiate.
- Pray and/or meditate.
- Find healing practices that work for you — and do them!
- Explore the arts and other expressive activities.

5

Cognitive Rewiring: Healing Our Minds with Activities and Games

Just fix my brain and I won't be crazy! (or dumb
or lazy or inappropriate...)
— Carolyn E. Dolen

You may say or think something like this every day. You know your
brain doesn't work right and you know that you can't act right until it
does. So this chapter explores how to "fix brains." Yes, it can happen!
Recent research shows brains can rewire after injury — if we work at it!

Chapter 3 "Brain Construction and Wiring" discusses how the brain
is originally wired. Here we explore what to repair and how to rewire
your brain and grow new cells to reconnect cognitively. We answer
questions about how we think and offer strategies, suggestions, activities,
and resources to improve communication skills. Topics include:

- Introduction: "dead" doesn't mean "gone"; new research.
- What is cognitive functioning? What needs to be fixed?
- What are typical cognitive problems?
- Can our cognitive connections improve? When? How?
- Activities/aids to improve cognitive functioning and learn skills.
- Survivor self-talk: How to "put in work orders to my brain."
- Rewiring activities: quiet and active, alone and with others.

Introduction

"Right, lady, heal my brain — as if it can be fixed — not! We all know that my brain injury short-circuited wires and fried connections. However mangled my brain cells, they're all I've got, so I'm going to protect them. Rest and relaxation is what I need. No newfangled experiments for my brain! The damage is done. Broken is broken and dead is dead."

Wait! "Dead" no longer applies to brain cells! The old scientific theory that all brain cells were distributed at birth and new ones didn't grow is itself dead! Findings of new tissue growth, even in older brains, put to rest that dinosaur thinking — and we're not talking about rat brains here, either! (Stein, Brailowsky, & Will, 1995).

How can we grow new brain cells? Stimulate your brain. Do anything other than veg out in front of the TV! Use your senses and get involved with life mentally, physically, spiritually, and socially. Beyond the utter logic of it, stimulating

> Words don't move mountains. Work, exacting work, moves mountains.
> — Danilo Dolci

body, mind, and spirit leads to a rich life. Yeah! Let's fix our brains! *I am living proof that we can fix our brains — we can continue to improve — if we work at it.*

What is cognitive functioning and what needs to be fixed?

Cognitive functioning is the way our brains see and process information to direct our actions. Because output is based on input received, the central thinking operation needs to be treated so we can observe and understand accurately to act properly. *"Fix my brain and I won't act crazy!"*

What problems are likely?

We can encounter problems with anything and everything that involves any thinking — even behaviors that used to be automatic, like dressing and bathing. More complex tasks that require us to remember and plan something can be a huge challenge!

Executive functioning. Trouble in this area is obvious to others as well as to us. This trouble comes as an inability to plan, organize, direct, and remember. This leads to deficits in problem solving, judgment, concept formation, processing speed, mental flexibility, and consistency. We also typically show a lack of ability to recognize our strengths and weaknesses; monitor, evaluate, and alter social behavior; screen out background noise; and make realistic vocational plans.

Attention and concentration. We frequently encounter problems with short-lived attention, straying off the task or conversation at hand. Are you sometimes criticized for not paying attention? Maybe it's because you can't hear somebody because of the background noise. We all seem to have an increased sensitivity to noise that others can just block out, which may explain our problems with crowds.

Why does our performance vary?
Are you frustrated at the unpredictability of your problems? Sometimes you can remember, then act competently — and other times you forget to tie your shoes? Brain injury does that!

Due to the nature of the damage, our ability to think and act varies a lot, but it's mostly because of our sensitivity to stress. If your current stress level is high — because of noise, inadequate sleep, or

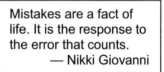

> Mistakes are a fact of life. It is the response to the error that counts.
> — Nikki Giovanni

nutrition, pain, medication issues, or other reasons — your abilities are greatly reduced. Basically, stress makes us stupid!

With all these deficit areas, can we get better?
Yes! Cognitive rehabilitation not only improves thinking ability, but also leads to significant overall improvement. Studies suggest that how well our intellectual and memory functions return affects our ultimate outcome, including our occupational outlook. Return to productive activity, success in the community, and even reentry to the work force is then possible. Most certainly, when we increase our cognitive skills, we are better able to emotionally adjust to, and maybe even accept, our injuries — partially because we're less disabled! To improve comes with a big "if," however — *if* we try!

What can survivors do to compensate for our deficits? Use SAFER!
Use the SAFER method, created by my wise counselor Dr. Christine Baser and me. Visualize SAFER on a stop sign: Stop, Assess, Fix, Examine, Retry. Remember when you were taught as a child to stop and look both ways before you crossed the street? This SAFER stop sign can remind you to cognitively override any problem when you feel confused or overloaded by a situation.

Rationale. Before you cross a street — in speaking or in our actions — first you need to stop what you're doing to assess the situation and develop a plan. Then you implement the plan to fix it. To determine if it works, you examine (test) the plan. If your plan doesn't work, you go back to the beginning to try again. If the new plan works, you proceed; if not, you stop again and develop another plan. You repeat this until you develop a strategy that works.

Note: There may be times when neither Plan A nor Plan B works. If Plans C and D also fail, perhaps it is best to try again another day. Sometimes the best plan may be to retreat. It doesn't mean you're quitting; it means you're smart enough to know when to regroup.

Personal experience. This SAFER plan reminds me of advice given by professional triathlete Mike Pigg at a training camp I attended, "Return home if you go for a bike ride and don't want to be there after a mile. For whatever reasons, your body doesn't want to ride at that time. Perhaps it needs to rest. Maybe you need to eat or desire another kind of exercise. Your body knows it doesn't want to ride, so listen to it and return home."

This works! Sometimes, inexplicably, I don't want to exercise or follow my workout plan. So, I alter it. Later, when I discover the reason, I'm glad I didn't push and make myself ill. Finally, after over 25 years, I'm getting it. Maybe in my next life it won't take me as long — which reminds me of a favorite anonymous quotation: "You keep getting what you're getting when you keep doing what you're doing."

How long will we keep improving?
As long as you work at it. "Use it or lose it" is especially appropriate for survivors. Even after several years, improvement in all areas has been

observed by professionals, caregivers, and, yes, even by survivors (Najenson, 1974). As your cognitive functioning improves, so does your emotional and behavioral functioning.

How can professionals help cognitive rehabilitation work?

Professionals know what to do and how to do it! They use methods that both rely on your strengths and acknowledge your weaknesses, so you don't do what doesn't work. These helpers teach you strategies to use to "do what you can with what you have." Special aids/devices are incorporated into your learning. You can use them after your formal cognitive rehabilitation time is finished.

Cognitive rehabilitation professionals include: speech-language pathologists/specialists, occupational therapists, and neuropsychologists. Other therapists may use cognitive skills in their work, too.

What are cognitive therapy goals and how are they achieved?

Because injury disorganized your brain and damaged your thinking abilities, your goals are to decrease disability and increase ability.

> Mind moves matter.
> — Virgil

The method is the same as fixing a broken connection: strengthen remaining areas, add new parts if needed, and rebuild so that work orders placed in your brain can be acted upon!

What are other cognitive connections?

Community colleges may offer classes specifically for brain-injury survivors, some including use of computer programs. Even if there is no designated class, general remedial classes work on skill deficits, too.

> A soul should always stand ajar, ready to welcome the ecstatic experience.
> — Emily Dickinson

Personal experience. When I was injured in 1976, there were no specific rehabilitation programs for survivors of brain injury. Because I knew I needed remedial help to regain my skills and there were no focused classes or therapies available, I enrolled in reading and study skills improvement classes at the local community college. Because of my previous degree in English education, the professors questioned why I was there. After hearing my reason, though, they encouraged me as I worked hard to rewire myself and relearn needed skills. Success!

Cognitive Connections at Home

Work at home? Yes! Your rewiring progress is much faster if you work wherever you are, whenever you can. Not everything you try will work, but doing nothing guarantees failure! "Keep knocking on doors."

Environmental Factors

Brains, like flowers, need air, water, light, and nutrients to bloom — plus appropriate music! — so you start with the environment. For success, you need to both reduce your disability and broaden your ability.

To reduce disability, because you're not able to screen out incidental sounds, you need learner-friendly music or white noise. Eliminate all other distracting noises — such as television, radio, or people talking — during work hours. Additionally, to recover from the overload, you usually need more rest and sleep than nondisabled others.

Personal experience. *I always play quiet music (usually Mozart or other classical) on my stereo when I work or drive. Music harmonizes my brain waves to help me focus on the task at hand and prevents me from developing road rage.*

Specific Survivor Needs

Figure out what your needs are
- **Timing.** Match activities, people, and places with the best time of day for you.
- **Medications.** Take them on time and in the right doses.
- **Food.** Choose how frequently to eat and what kinds of food. Make sure you take vitamin and mineral supplements to help your rewiring.
- **Activity.** Find the right amount and frequency of activity for you. Appropriate exercise is crucial.
- **Sleep/rest.** Learn what amount of sleep at night and rest periods during the day are best for you.

Personal experience. *After over 30 years of a lot of trial and error, I learned that certain food, sleep, exercise, and other lifestyle needs are essential to my health. I no longer apologize for them — they just are the way they are!*

My daily needs include sleep (between 9-10 hours per night), food (fresh fruit/yogurt/cereal for breakfast; sandwich, apple, and dark chocolate for lunch; a snack pre- and post-exercise; protein, rice, heaping salads and/or other fresh vegetables for dinner; and a bedtime snack), exercise (minimum of 1 to 1½ hours, which always includes yoga or stretching), and music (whenever I'm indoors or in my car).

My daily lifestyle needs include lots of time outdoors eating, working, and playing (preferably near or in the ocean), relaxed sit-down dining, bicycle rides, gardening/yard work, plenty of light, a variable and usually slow pace, visits with friends, and interaction with other friendly folks.

My favorite activities are running on the beach, jumping in the ocean as a reward, cycling along the coast, and greeting kids of all ages everywhere! Weekly needs include two weight-training sessions, a music and/or improv rehearsal, church participation, a lengthy telephone talk with my adopted sister in Minnesota, and email visits with assorted friends around the country and world. I also used to see a psychotherapist on a weekly basis. Bi-weekly or monthly, I see my acupuncturist, chiropractor, massage therapist, and talk with my Cape Cod brother.

Also, because I learned that noise short-circuits my brain (especially trains, trucks, traffic, barking dogs, honking horns), I avoid crowds and warehouse stores. I ask not to be disturbed before 9 AM or after 9 PM at home. If any of these

> Mistakes are part of life. It is the response to error that counts.
> — Nikki Giovanni

factors occur, it's not healthy for anyone! (After reading this, I think I sound like an ocean creature! Maybe in another life...)

Environmental Suggestions

- **Place.** Your learning location needs to be quiet, adequately lighted, and peaceful.

- **Background.** Play special music or run a fan to block out distracting bursts of noise. Turn off the TV and talk-radio. Ask people to talk elsewhere.
- **Light.** Use natural or good-quality artificial light.
- **Time.** Use whatever is your optimal time of day. Mornings, when we are fresh after a good night's sleep, are usually best — but not too early. Sometime after 9 or 10 AM usually works. Most of us tend to fade or fatigue in the early evening.
- **Pace.** Slow and unhurried with frequent breaks. Plan activities to include rest/quiet periods during the day. Alternating more active and less active days can be helpful.

Survivor Strategies to Improve Cognitive Functioning

- **Use all your senses.** Say, hear, see, and do — to reinforce memory.
- **Use positive self-talk.** "Good!" "That's it!" "You're getting it!"
- **Use a calendar and notebook.** Log important information such as appointments, birthdays, etc. Or use a "Day-Timer," "brain-in-a-binder," etc.
- **Do puzzles.** Sudoku puzzles stimulate your brain, re-establish logic patterns, and improve visual tracking. They're fun, too!
- **Spend time alone.** Plan your time alone and share your experiences later — or not!

> It's not what you've got; it's what you use that makes a difference.
> — Zig Ziglar

Prosthetic Memory Devices

Now we're talking! Electronic brains to the rescue! Everyone else uses a variety of brain boosters — day planners, calendars, checklists, and computers — in their daily lives. Let's use memory devices to help us return to productive work — and maybe even the work force!

Return to work with a memory deficit? Pulleeeez! Survivors need something more sophisticated than a calendar in order to perform at our former jobs. How about using a computer

> Do what you can, with what you have, where you are.
> — Teddy Roosevelt

program that provides a structure for work tasks? Research studies have found these programs to be especially useful cognitive orthotic devices (Parente, 1991). See *Brain Injury Rewiring for Loved Ones* for information on electronic memory aids and computer tools.

Games

Play a game to learn or practice a skill. *It works for me!* Modifying rules, such as teaming, improve chances for both fun and success. Different skills are needed, so you'll be sure to find something that suits you.

- **Electronic games.** Both video and computer games are fun. Stick with ones that teach you skills that you need. *First person shooter games are not a good idea.*
- **Table games.** Anything you enjoy! See *Brain Injury Rewiring for Loved Ones* for ideas.
- **Word and number games.** Word Find, Sudoku, etc.
- **Manual games.** Ping-Pong, pool, Foos Ball, etc.
- **Life!** Virtually anything, including chores, can be a game!

Self-Talk for Survivors

What you say to yourself — your self-talk — is even more important than what is said by others. Although positive self-talk is seen as a helpful strategy for emotional health, I also rely on it as a cognitive tool. Why? Because nothing is automatic anymore! As my friend Cheryl Burns described it, *"I need to put in work orders to my brain"* before it will carry out a task.

Uses of Self-Talk

Not only can self-talk be used in stressful situations, e.g., driving, presenting, or going somewhere new, but it can also be used at home when doing physical or mental work. Self-talk is also helpful in recreational pursuits or when learning a new activity. Especially useful in social situations, self-talk — silent, obviously! — is best if done immediately afterward to keep the interchange freshly in mind.

When learning a new activity or correcting a mistake.
Positive phrases that give direction are a good way to instruct others —
why not use them on yourself? Examples include: "What I need to do
now is…", "OK, that's not what you want here. What you need to do
is…", and "Now, let's try it again. You can do it!" I also say, "Come on!"
a lot to motivate myself, especially when doing a challenging physical
activity.

   *Personal experience. This kind of interchange was used many times
the summer I learned to surf at the age of 48 — and it worked! I am now
surfing — not always successfully or with real surfers out on the big
waves, but I am surfing. As my coach Kahuna Bob used to say, "The best
surfer is the one who has the most fun!"*

   When a minor mistake is made, if you say, "Oops!" or "Shoot!"
instead of curse words, you apply the same forgiveness and acceptance to
yourself that you ask of others. Are you not as worthy?

As a self-esteem aid.
"Fix my brain and I won't be crazy" is not only about your brain
working; it's related to your self-esteem. To feel okay about yourself, you
need a functioning control center. When you give yourself directions to
do those things that are no longer automatic, you provide the structure to
complete a task. In so doing, you feel good about yourself, regardless of
the size of the task. *I still give myself directions over thirty years later
and my self-esteem is quite healthy!*

As a memory aid.
Self-talk works on your nearly universal memory impairment —
especially auditory. When you speak, listen, and then do something, your
senses are totally focused on the task at hand. No extraneous thoughts or
feelings or other people or things distract you.

   To hear yourself repeat something also reinforces what you said and
helps you understand what you need to do. Talking oneself through any
task requires more interactive functioning of the brain than if something
is done automatically. Actions are intentional and nothing is left out.

In social or stressful situations.

You can remind yourself that the situation is something you can handle. It is reassuring to hear comforting words, especially when they come from someone you know has your best interest at heart, in this case, yourself!

> The greater danger for most of us is not that our aim is too high and we miss it, but that it is too low and we reach it.
> — Michelangelo

Kinds of Self-Talk

The phrase "words can hurt and words can heal" applies to your self-talk. You have the power to help or harm yourself every minute of the day. What you choose to say to yourself — both aloud and in your mind — can, to a large extent, determine how you feel about yourself.

Positive self-talk.

Hearing an encouraging voice is helpful any time, but it is vital when planning or doing some task. *I use the words, "Okay, good" or "All right, good" with myself a lot because I'm telling myself that*

> You wouldn't eat garbage, why put it in your head?
> — Ann Landers

everything is okay, I did well, and I'll do well on the next task. It's as though I'm re-parenting myself, which I actually am — I am creating a new person. On your journey, you only want to carry what is useful in your backpack — nothing that is unnecessary or bogs you down.

Negative self-talk.

This kind of self-talk just reinforces a poor self-image — that you're inadequate, no good, not worthy, etc. Pessimistic talk also elicits those negative feelings that lie just under your surface — the ones you continually fight as you climb your mountain. Replacing disapproving words — and profanities — with non-judgmental words such as "Oops!" is so much better for your psyche and lightens your backpack.

 Personal experience. *I used to use a lot of negative self-talk — until 1988 when I enrolled in a course that was part of a Master's program at San Diego State University.*

One of the requirements for Dr. Tom McKenzie's "Behavior Change in Sport and Physical Education" was to select a personal behavior that each student didn't like, monitor it, and develop a technique to change it. I chose negative self-talk — mostly a string of profanities uttered in frequent rage at my failures. Dr. McKenzie loaned me a counter that was worn like a wristwatch.

Unfortunately — or fortunately! — it was easy to use to keep track. I remember how disturbed I was that first morning to see that by 8 AM I'd already uttered nearly 20 profanities! Needless to say, my mood was also affected by this negativity, so I vowed to change.

What was my method? Count profanities, track the time, and, if necessary, add a punishment — snapping a rubber band on my wrist. Usually, just the act of counting was sufficient for me to stop doing it. Early morning and evening were the most troublesome. For many of us, these times are the most fragile and difficult periods of the day — we've either not really begun our day or we're ready to retire.

Part of the process was to submit a paper detailing my plan — including a reward system that was based on degree of accomplishment of the goal. For me, merely reducing negative self-talk and improving my mood and self-image was reward enough, so I didn't need anything else! My smile was reward enough! In the nearly twenty years since this life-changing experience I can't say that I don't occasionally utter a profanity or feel down on myself. But what I can say is that I no longer utter a string of curses. Now I give myself directions about what needs to be changed; I also say, "Okay, good!" a lot.

Word choice

The best words to use are "need," "want," "not need," and "not want" because they are unemotional words. Any emotionally loaded phrases are guaranteed to sidetrack the task at hand. Corrections need to be offered in a positive manner. Of course, enthusiastic praise — given anytime — improves chances for success.

Activities to Improve Cognitive Connections

Challenging your brain stimulates brain growth, builds brain circuitry, and rewires your cognitive connections to be able to reconnect with the world. Involvement with others is the first step toward moving away from the egocentricity (self-centeredness) that is inevitable after a traumatic sickness or injury. Another reward is that interacting is fun!

Quiet activities.
- Listen to music.
- Meditate.
- Do word games, mazes, crossword puzzles.
- Play board/card games.
- Play a musical instrument/take lessons.
- Assemble jigsaw puzzles.
- Design puzzles or games.
- Assemble or design models to keep, sell, or donate.
- Paint or draw. Consider starting with paint-by-number kits.
- Sew or knit.
- Keep a diary in written or audio form.
- Write stories or poems to keep, share, or submit for publication.
- Watch selected television programs.
- Arrange or rearrange your family photo album.
- Sing — along with radio, tapes, CDs — anything!
- Make crafts or do woodwork to keep, donate, or sell.

Activities that require more energy.
- Visit a museum, zoo, or nature preserve.
- Play a musical instrument — anything!
- Sing along with music or in a musical group.
- Attend concerts, lectures, theater.
- Photograph.
- Sculpt with clay or another medium.
- Join an improvisation comedy workshop.
- Exercise/stretch — do anything!
- Walk — indoors or out.

- Practice yoga.
- Dance, especially a challenging activity like ballet, tap, or square dancing.
- Join a Toastmasters' group.
- Garden — indoors or out.
- Videotape an activity or series of activities.
- Take a class-in anything!
- Build anything!

Not good ideas.
Playing video games or similar computer-based games is not a good choice because very limited parts of the brain are used for many of the games. Shooter games are especially bad in this regard. You need to rewire your whole brain into a normal pattern — video games do not do this.

Vegging out with the TV is also not a good idea. Why? It reminds you that you are an outsider and reaffirms a sense of helplessness, worthlessness, and social isolation. Need any more reasons? Okay, one more — it doesn't help your brain function get better.

Work-related activities.
- Do computer activities. Taking surveys on-line is fun.
- Read and underline articles in newspapers, magazines, books.
- Label all cupboards, drawers, closets by listing contents.
- Design and build cars, planes, toys.
- Cook, bake, or learn how — donate or sell products.
- Plan an outing using maps and train or bus schedules.

Work activities.
- Care for animals.
- Refinish and/or repair furniture.
- Design and build furniture or toys.
- Construct/maintain a compost/worm bin.
- Repair/recycle household items/small appliances.
- Auto or motorcycle detailing/repair.
- Bicycle/skateboard repair.

- Yard work; snow shoveling.
- Wash windows for businesses.
- Carpentry/construction or picture framing.
- Pet care or pet boarding.
- Babysitting, elder sitting, respite care.
- Computer data entry; web site design and maintenance
- Housecleaning.
- Home repair.
- Start a business!

Caution about running a business.
A friend of mine who is a successful business owner says that running a business is difficult for *nondisabled* people. Many business functions not related to the primary activity are too taxing for survivors. Set yourself up for success by partnering with someone who can and will do the tasks that might be difficult and/or draining, e.g., accounting, bill collection, preparing tax returns and other reports, and marketing.

Cognitive Connection Checklist

As a final word on cognitive connections, here's a list to make sure you are doing everything you can.

Brain enhancers.
- Nutritious diet.
- Mental and physical activity, especially aerobic exercise.
- Sleep and rest.
- Meditation.
- Music.
- Light.
- Positive self-talk.
- Nurturing people and places.
- Creative pursuits.

Brain nutrients.
- Five to seven daily servings of fruits and veggies — a serving is usually 1/2 cup.

- Two to three servings of protein — 1/2 gram per pound of body weight per day. Eat "brain food" — oily fish — at least twice weekly.
- Six to ten daily servings of whole unprocessed grains.
- Drink water — 1/2 ounce per pound of body weight per day.
- Daily multivitamin.
- A nutritious diet provides electrolytes such as calcium, magnesium, and potassium for tissue vitality and repair.

Balance.
- Input and output.
- Activity and rest.
- Food and water.
- Mental and physical activity.
- Quiet and busy time.
- Alone and social time.

Brain poisons.
- Nicotine.
- Saturated and trans fats.
- Sugars.
- Stress.
- Junk food — fatty, salty, sugary.
- Alcohol and street drugs.
- Inactivity.

> *Remember: "Garbage in, garbage out."*

Summary

"Put work orders in your brain," "Use it or lose it!" Remember that mistakes are part of life. It is your response to error that counts (Nikki Giovanni).

Here are other lessons from this chapter:

- Use SAFER — Stop, Assess, Fix, Examine, Retry — to solve problems.
- Log important information on a calendar and in a notebook or use a Day-Timer, brain-in-a-binder, etc.
- Use all your senses — say, hear, see, do — to reinforce memory.
- Do Sudoku and other puzzles to stimulate your brain, re-establish logic patterns, and improve visual tracking. *And they're fun!*
- Learn your needs: best time of day (for activities, people, and places), food (how frequently and what kinds of food), activity (amount, frequency, and duration), and sleep/rest (amount and when).

> Often we look so long at the closed door that we don't see the one that has opened for us.
> — Patricia Neal

- Spend time alone.
- Set up your environment for success using music, light, plants, etc.
- Eat a healthful, nutritious diet.
- Exercise — mentally and physically — every day.
- Do not veg out in front of the TV.
- Avoid video games.
- Know that you can fix your brain — if you work at it!
- Use positive and encouraging self-talk: "Good!" "That's it!" "You're getting it!" "Let's go!"

6
Emotional Rewiring: Healing Our Feelings and Spirits

It isn't for the moment you are stuck that you need courage, but for the long, uphill climb back to sanity and faith and security.
— Anne Morrow Lindbergh

You survived the trauma. Now your real ascent begins. No more practice climbing walls — your mountain is in the real world. *It looks much steeper than I remember, and I don't see the top yet, encumbered with my beat-up backpack with its fraying seams and sticking zippers. Formerly colored "vintage burgundy," now my backpack looks more like last week's Ripple — complete with storied stains and smells. Its special scent is moldy-apple, rancid-sunflower-seed, and shriveled-raisin trail mix. Its waterproof coating is long gone, replaced by a gnarly surface that grabs every thorn along the path. This old worn pack looks light and easy to carry — but isn't. If I can just reach the next level of this mountain, maybe I'll meet another angel — is this the part where "God helps those who help themselves?"*

Introduction

To empower your climbing success, you need to set yourself up to succeed by lightening your load. You inspect your backpack for damage, clean and repack it with the appropriate gear. It's the same way you prepare for other trips, except this expedition is a life journey — and it's one-way. Let's inspect your emotional baggage to see what changes you need to make for a successful climb — however far you may go.

This chapter explores some ways people deal with grief and loss. Interspersed throughout are numerous personal experiences from my own recovery journey. Topics include:

- Grief and loss: stages of grief and dimensions of loss.
- Mourning rites and memorial services.
- Bereavement.
- Similarities among survivors.
- Substance use and abuse.
- Emotional issues and what to do to facilitate the journey.

Grief and Loss

Healing from emotional injury is similar to mending from physical injury, as my first psychologist and one of my best angels, DJ, explained to me.

As with other wounds, the first step is to clean out debris that retards and prevents healing, so the wound is flushed. If it is infected, it may need to be scrubbed until it bleeds. You may say, "Don't I hurt enough? Why cause myself more pain?" I argued this, too, until DJ reminded me how I cut on myself! Enduring this pain is easier if you understand that it leads to healing. With no cleansing, there is no mending.

How do you cleanse? First, you must grieve your loss. Are you thinking, "I didn't die, so what exactly is lost?"

The way things used to be is gone forever. Life may look the same on the surface, but on deeper levels, the person you were — that self — is lost, both to you and to your loved ones. Missing along with that self are the vital roles and

> The art of living lies less in eliminating our troubles than in growing with them.
> — Bernard Baruch

interests that identified who that self was, e.g., career, hobbies, and family/social positions.

What is grief?

Grief is a journey. It is an ancient pilgrimage, yet a fresh one for all who embark on it. No one can avoid it. While everyone takes the same trip, it is different for each of us, as you go at your own pace and in your own way. You cannot escape it — you must go through it — sometimes several times. And you must do it yourself — no one can do it for you.

Grief is work. It is difficult and seemingly endless. But if you don't work through it after a loss, no healing or emotional growth can occur. As with all work, there are stages of grief.

Stages of Grief: The Grief Cycle

If you understand the grief cycle that everyone experiences after a tragic loss, it helps you to cope with yours. Elizabeth Kübler-Ross and other well-known grief experts theorize that people travel through the following stages on the grief journey:

- Denial and isolation.
- Anger.
- Bargaining.
- Depression.
- Acceptance.

The first three stages are attempts to overcome the loss — with or without complete awareness of it. The last two stages are reactions and responses to the loss. Much of the following discussion is based on Kübler-Ross's work in her book *On Death and Dying* (1969).

First Stage: Denial and Isolation

Denial — "It can't be!" — replaces the initial shock of what happened. Then, as you feel the sting of reality's slap, the next stage — isolation — follows. *Does "Leave me alone!" sound familiar?* People are often similar to hurt animals: you curl up and hibernate until it's all better. However, in this case, there's a problem with the natural response — it won't be all better.

How quickly and easily you pass through this stage is determined by your character, which defense mechanisms you used before the injury, and your insight compared to the amount you are told.

What is denial?
"I do not want to believe in what I see I can't do." You may notice diminished capacity, but you may place blame on the activity, people, day, weather — anything but you. You simply cannot painlessly lose such a valued part of who you are!

Closely allied with denial as defense mechanisms are escape and avoidance, common strategies for everyone — disabled or not. Some escape with drugs or alcohol to reduce the feeling of loss. Others avoid a particular activity. Still others attempt — through endless classes, study, and effort — to regain what they have lost.

What to do.
Exercise healthy muscles to benefit injured ones. Perhaps a positive part of denial is that some survivors try to strengthen other aspects of their bodies, minds, or personalities in the hope that the weak part will somehow grow stronger, too. It works!

Because denying reality takes a lot of psychological time and energy, it's not necessarily a bad idea since that buys you time. To enable you to make realistic plans for your loss, you need time to fully understand it.

Second Stage: Anger or Rage

When the "No, it's not true!" stage cannot be maintained any longer, it is replaced by feelings of anger, rage, envy, and resentment. "No, it didn't happen" gives way to "Yes, it happened to me, but — why me?" These expressions of anger are natural. In fact, anger is your longest-lasting response to your injury.

You transfer your anger in any and all directions and project it onto the environment — and whoever is in the way — in ways that seem random and out of proportion to the offense. Everyone is at fault for everything and nobody can do anything right. *Does this sound familiar?* This stage is especially difficult for your loved ones to cope with — those closest to you are often the targets of the rage.

What to do.
Be aware and try to control your anger — for everyone's sakes! Remember to use the SAFER method — Stop, Asses, Fix, Examine, and

Retry — when something angers you, so you do not alienate the very people who are trying their best to help you.

Third Stage: Bargaining

Helpful for brief periods of time, this stage attempts to postpone or reduce the effects of the loss. It also includes a prize for good behavior and usually sets a self-imposed deadline — "Please, just one more..." Usually these bargains are attempted with God — "If you fix me, I'll dedicate myself to the church/temple, etc." They can also be made with significant others or hospital staff — "If you use your scientific expertise to cure me, I'll..." Who hasn't attempted to improve a bad situation with a promise to do better next time? — "If you let me do..., then I'll..." The positive aspects of this stage are that you're highly motivated, enthusiastic about therapy, and willing to work.

What to do.
Remain hopeful in order to stay motivated and keep working hard. It's better to make some progress than to expect huge or unrealistic improvements. Think "small steps for success."

Fourth Stage: Depression

Anger that has turned inward becomes depression. By this stage, a sense of great loss and hopelessness replaces denial, outward anger, and bargaining. Hope changes to despair. You may say, "It's useless to try anymore. Nothing works." Depression is a normal and natural reaction not just to a stressful and

> Life is not always what one wants it to be, but to make the best of it as it is, is the only way of being happy.
> — Jennie Jerome Churchill

traumatic event, but also to the devastation of the injury. How depressed you feel depends on both the size of the loss and the value that you placed on what you lost.

Following a severe life disappointment, e.g., a job loss, divorce, or death of someone close, people typically experience situational depression. After a brain injury, however, survivors are commonly diagnosed with clinical depression, which is more severe.

What to do.
If you're not interested in anything that used to bring you joy, continually want to be alone, sleep all the time, and/or feel suicidal, seek professional help before it gets worse. Also see "Specific Helpful Behaviors" near the end of this chapter.

Fifth Stage: Acceptance

Although acceptance is the goal of the grieving process, it is not an end point. Even if you reach this stage, you may never stop grieving. Acceptance is a time of adjustment and adaptation, not necessarily a happy one. You may say, "Okay, this is it — this is what I have to work with. I'll make the most of it and turn the lemons into lemonade. I know that those who accept their disability aren't depressed or ill, and they don't act disturbed. So, how can it happen?"

In fits and starts — just like the rest of your rehabilitation. One day an "Aha" experience may occur — or not. Either way, if you keep working to improve and stay/get involved with the community in social and productive ways, it'll happen, sooner or later.

Acceptance is the first step to action. It does not mean tolerating nor does it mean doing nothing. It means working with what is left, rather than wishing it weren't so — which makes it difficult to learn. At this stage, you're often very motivated and actively seek improvement. Rehabilitation focuses on strengthening some abilities, compensating for others, and adapting the environment.

> God grant me the serenity to accept the things I cannot change, the courage to change the things that I can, and the wisdom to know the difference.
> — Serenity Prayer

Personal experience. *I learned the following lessons from my grief journey.*

- There is no order to this journey, but acceptance is the last stop.
- There is no predictable time to spend at any one stage.

- Some stages may be visited more than once.
- Sometimes several stages are engaged at the same time.
- You may favor one stage over others — and return again and again when stressed. *Anger is my "favorite."*
- Frequently anger is intermingled with any or all of the other stages other than acceptance.
- You may repeat the entire cycle again and again whenever you experience another major loss.
- You may seem to arrive at acceptance, but the visit may be short.
- Acceptance may take 15-20 years to achieve — or it may never be reached. *It took me nearly 19 years to feel any degree of acceptance beyond resignation. Now I remember to remind myself: "God doesn't make junk!"*

Dimensions of Loss

As you move through the various stages of the grief cycle after your injury, you notice that parts of your life are missing. Because not facing a loss can lead to self-destructive behaviors, it's vital that you look at those missing parts. What is absent? There are five distinct kinds of loss: loss of a significant person/valued other, loss of an external object, developmental loss, loss of security, and loss of some aspect of self (Tanner, 1984). In the following discussion, broadly based on this work, you'll focus on your losses.

Loss of significant person/valued other.
Brain injury results in the "death" of the former person. Although your name is the same, you're different. Your previous self is lost — not only to yourself, but also to your family and friends; as if you were dead. Without speech, and the words necessary to describe wants, feelings, hopes, thoughts, attitudes, and beliefs, you have a feeling of separation.

Loss of external object and/or abilities.
These losses may not be felt immediately. Naturally, the value of an object or ability determines the extent of the loss — the more you valued something, the stronger you feel the impact of its loss.

Personal experience. *Even now, decades later, every time I see an MG, I fondly recall my cute little 1968 cherry-red MG Midget with removable black hardtop, wood and leather interior, spinner hubs, luggage rack...*

Often the symbolic value you placed on these objects causes the most grief. Not only does seeing an old friend (*like my car*) bring out tremendous sadness, it also provokes a grief reaction for a missing object by reminding you of your lost abilities. Seeing old trophies or sports equipment could cause pain to former athletes or instruments to musicians or carpentry and drawing tools to woodworkers and artists.

You may greet a thoughtful gesture by a friend, e.g., bringing tools to add to your collection, by exploding with anger or tears. See the "Last Rites" and "Memorial Service" sections later in this chapter for ways to deal with this loss.

Developmental loss.

Usually gradual in nature and associated with growth and aging, this loss is considered to be the least significant. Most adults experience some degree of mid-life crisis in middle age. At milestone-birthdays like 40 or 50, they face the reality that, perhaps, some — or many — of their youthful hopes and dreams, e.g. becoming a Hollywood star or famous athlete or saving the world from any number of ills, may not be achieved in this lifetime.

As natural as the aging process is, the suddenness of the losses — like a tire blowing out on the freeway — is what causes the sorrow. This instant aging immediately halts your progression toward achieving your goals, however farfetched they may be. Not that it totally derails all chances of fulfilling youthful hopes and dreams — that is up to God and each person. You can also alter some goals. But the injury will be at least a temporary roadblock on your highway to the stars or wherever.

Loss of security.

Your injury has replaced knowing what to expect with unpredictability of just about everything. The rules of the game as you knew them have changed; nothing is known for sure anymore and you become increasingly aware that your former lifestyle will not and cannot continue.

Financial insecurity is an especially heavy burden for those survivors who previously supported themselves or a family. The good feelings that came from providing for financial needs are replaced by high anxiety and despair over how to pay for the high costs associated with all the health services that are now required.

Personal experience. One of my saddest memories was that terrible day when I awakened with the dreadful thought of "I wonder what I will discover I can't do today."

Loss of some aspect of self.

This is the greatest loss and covers all the aspects of your being. You are less than you were — intellectually, emotionally, and physically. Not wanting to depress anyone, I won't remind you of these changes in detail — you know what you lost.

> What I was, I am not.
> What I was, I am never going to be again.
> — Maureen Campbell-Korves

Personal experience. Knowing that my physical skills were impaired, friends of my parents brought books — everybody knew our family loved the written word! Sadly, they didn't know my cognitive skills were impaired, too — the books were too complex, so I ignored them. My parents were upset and confused that I didn't like to read anymore. I did like to read — I just couldn't read difficult material. Short stories with only one or two characters were all I could handle — children's books were my favorites. Imagine my folks' feelings when their daughter, the English teacher, could only read simple material! "Has she lost her intellectual capacity? The tests said she was still smart. Why doesn't she act like it? What's wrong with her? Maybe she's just not trying!" Their responses showed yet another painful result of inaccurate and incomplete testing.

What about your family?

They lost a lot, too. Loved ones may feel grief and loss, either indirectly through empathy with you or directly because of your changed relationship, lifestyle, and dreams. Understand that anger is part of

> The more sympathy you give, the less you need.
> — Malcolm S. Forbes

their grief process, just as it is part of yours. Siblings probably won't like that the balance of the family changed with the injury. Roles are different now and more may be asked of them. They want it to be the way it was, too.

If your blood-related family doesn't work, create one that does! Adopt new sisters and brothers, even parents, into a group of your design. In this win-win situation, several good things can happen: the load is shared, guilt is reduced, and able and willing others can play important roles in your life, either temporarily or permanently. Although "family" is usually considered to be those people who are blood relatives, "kin" can mean any group of people who are related by a common belief or goal such as love for one another or for something bigger.

Personal experience. Unfortunately, my family did not participate in therapy with me. To this day, I do not know if they went on their own. But I doubt it because of their personalities and the culture of the time. Due to physical and/or emotional distance, my two brothers and my parents were not able to be involved or provide the supportive environment I needed — both pre- and post-injury. But they did what they could and I was not totally abandoned. Inherited character traits rose to the challenge, and my new best friend Marlys — really, my first angel — took over the key-person role. In my family's defense, there was little awareness about TBI during the 1970s, so my family did not know what I needed or where to go for assistance.

So, while research clearly demonstrates the importance of family to recovery, I am testimony that recovery can occur with little more than a gifted gene pool and strong family values. Did I mention the hand of God?

Mourning Rites and Memorial Services

Psychologists used to think that the best way to recover from the death of a loved one was to eliminate reminders. Attitudes about grieving are different these days.

Psychological Benefits of Grieving

Grief experts now encourage mourners to include memorial ceremonies in their grief work because remembering validates what is lost and liberates the griever to move on. By affirming the loss, an official ceremony also affirms to all the importance of a worthy replacement.

> When a person is born, we rejoice, and when they're married, we jubilate, but when they die, we try to pretend that nothing happened.
> — Margaret Mead

Just as cleaning a wound enables it to heal, so you need to express your sorrow for your losses before you can regain a sense of order in your new life as you reclaim control and purpose by rewiring.

Personal and familial grieving methods may differ, but they are all valid. I hope that you and your loved ones are inspired by the wide variety of mourning rites and funeral customs throughout the world to create your own memorial service so you can mourn together. Let's explore how some religions and cultures build healing rituals into their mourning processes.

Jewish rites.

In traditional Judaism, mourners sit *shivah* (Hebrew for "seven"), dedicating a whole week to remembering the departed one. Other temple members prepare and deliver meals to the bereaved, who are directed to stay home, not work, and not do anything pleasurable. Mourners who have experienced this believe that it is grief at its deepest and find it helpful to have the time to focus, to release the deep feelings in a safe place, and to get it all out. Catharsis renews body, mind, and spirit.

Catholic wakes.
The Irish wake was traditionally the center of all funeral customs. It is a public recognition of grief, a collective tribute to the dead, and also a social event. In the past, friends and families of the deceased gathered in one room of a wake house, sharing sympathy, stories, and beverages. Another room was reserved for praying near the body.

Samoan rites.
In the tradition of the Samoan culture, family and friends gather at a luau to both remember a loved one and mark a time to move on with their lives. At a *faluela* celebration, loved ones listen to music, eat food, and engage in favorite activities of the one who died. Such events may also raise scholarship funds to honor the fallen one.

Non-denominational memorial services.
A television program about the life of a survivor showed another way to deal with grief. Out of frustration, the injured boy said he wanted to bury all of the old trophies, pictures, uniforms, and equipment that no longer represented him because he was tired of everyone recalling his former superior athletic abilities. His family participated in the service and burial, and then celebrated the new boy who had come to live with them. *Sounds like the phoenix rising from the ashes, doesn't it?*

This idea offers potential healing for everyone, particularly when a younger person is severely injured and has little likelihood of recovering his former skills. For those survivors who still love the same activities and have some ability to do them, the service could be more symbolic and spoken, with partial rather than total destruction of memorabilia to provide closure and validation for what was lost — for everyone.

Some survivors may need a concrete way to express grief, like burying or burning, if they prefer hands-on activities or if other typical ways are inadequate, says survivor and author Kate Vincent (1989).

Plan for the void.
What was lost may be more meaningful than anyone realized. Your own response may surprise you. When you and your loved ones communicate your feelings, though, other alternatives can be revealed, such as

incorporating your former aim into a new goal. If there is a realistic — and spoken — plan to fill the void with something of equal value, energy goes toward a new goal rather than mourning the old one — ignoring "the elephant in the living room." *I often wonder how a memorial service could have eased my grieving — and that of my family, too.*

Personal experience. For me, sadness came not from others' reminiscences but from mine, so burying everything would have been worse than having no service at all, since much of what I treasured would be gone. Whether others remembered or not, nothing was said, as was proper behavior then. And, because survivors don't get subtleties, I never knew of others' feelings except by the pained expression on their faces and their avoidance of activity — and me. I recall thinking, "I wish somebody would say something!" I wanted to share my grief — and discuss realistic alternatives and other activities I valued to fill the void from my losses.

I learned something from my experience that I've never forgotten: To not deny a loss — to be open to others' grief, to be available to listen, and to actively help them do their grief work. I also decided to risk saying or doing something that might offend them as I tried to help them grieve. By ignoring their important loss, others ignore them, then they feel even more alone. I can help them lighten and carry their backpacks.

Final Note

Survivors' responses to a survey I used in my thesis demonstrated the value of the memorial service. Although the questions were specific to recovery, many survivors included all the details about their injuries — from a victim's perspective! I

> The best way to get a new part in life's play is to stop rehearsing the past.
> — Noel ben Shea

purposely didn't ask "what happened?" because that information is not helpful to others and I don't do "victim." This showed me what happens to survivors who don't experience a final good-bye to their previous selves. Those respondents were stuck in the past — although it doesn't take a brain injury for this to occur. Ask anyone who has attended a 10- or 20- or 30-year high school reunion!

Bereavement

If you consider that "time heals all wounds," is it a surprise that difficulties adjusting to loss relate to the lack of acceptable time to grieve? Not only has the tone of modern life affected the quality of "permissible" bereavement, but the speed. Acceptable American grieving time decreased from three years in 1927 to six months in 1950 to the week or so decreed by Amy Vanderbilt in 1972. Today, most American companies establish three days as the official grieving period. In some countries, the mourning period has been entirely abolished.

Typical length of time
Some studies suggest that six to twelve months is the typical and acceptable length of time required to grieve a major loss, depending on the awareness of the people involved and the significance of the loss or losses (Tanner, 1984).

I submit it is far longer than that. No one with whom I've ever spoken who experienced significant loss reached acceptance sooner than a couple of years — and many years is the norm. Clinicians agree. Recent studies suggest that for some people, mourning could last a lifetime, especially when they see daily reminders of their loss.

"There is no rule of thumb for the length of time it will take to grieve trauma. And whether there is any therapeutic intervention, and how much, may affect the degree of acceptance" (Isenhart, 1994).

Why so long to acceptance?
Is it because there is no actual loss of a physical body, even though what is gone may be as profound and grief inducing for the survivor? For social beings, if society does not validate the loss, it is far worse — another reason for support groups.

Sometimes people will go through an acceptance stage only to be thrust back into another stage — usually anger — because of another trauma. Is acceptance related to degree of awareness?

Higher-functioning survivors.
Several researchers suggest that this group may both experience a greater loss and demonstrate more distress. Others likely agree with the studies

showing that we typically experience more emotional distress than those with greater disability and perceive our loss of abilities more acutely than lower-functioning survivors (Prigatano, 1987; Kay, 1986). Some psychologists suggest that this may arise out of frustration at attempts to resume life as it was pre-injury and as we struggle with hidden or subtle deficits — when we look fine, but aren't fine. Researchers also found that we may experience a greater sense of loss in pre-injury roles, lifestyle, and employment status (Hendryx, 1989; Kay, 1986).

Increased awareness leads to increased denial, complicating the loss issue. It may seem to be a mutually exclusive response — the more I know, the more I don't want to know. Or it could be that we are more aware of our losses, especially as we progress in our recovery. Sometimes, the more we have gained, the more we *see* that we have lost.

Personal experience. Unfortunately, I still frequently misunderstand nuances — usually when I think I have made a breakthrough! Whether it's someone I want to impress, such as an employer or just my smart friends, I think, "Yes! I'm relating and actually understanding!"

Then there is a thud — when I run headlong into that lurking cloud that at times looks as easy to walk through as a sheet of mist but acts like a wall of steel. Because gray mist and steel are the same color may be one reason I'm deceived. Another may be that perhaps I do get it for an instant, just not long enough to fully comprehend. I still try, and at least now I see more mist than steel.

Long-term survivors.
There may be more sensitivity, distress, irritability, restlessness, and tiredness as time from injury increases, according to research. This results in psychosocial, and/or work-related problems in addition to developing substance abuse problems, particularly alcohol dependence (Cobble et al., 1991; Thomsen, 1984; Kreutzer et al., 1996). The cumulative weight of the emotional struggle and the tremendous energy costs of continuous rehabilitation could account for this — but don't despair. Simple awareness of this phenomenon can help us to accept, adapt, and develop new strategies! *I often think of my initial psych-ward-or-suicide prognosis, and feel better.*

Similarities among Survivors

Just as there are many similarities among survivors with regard to age, gender, education, employment history, and lifestyle immediately before the injury, there are personality similarities, too.

> It is not only the kind of injury that matters, but the kind of head.
> — Sir Charles Symonds

Although most people find joy in everyday occurrences, and laughter — internal jogging — is crucial for repair, have you noticed that we survivors don't laugh much? Why? In 1995 my former therapist, Dr. Christine Baser, suggested that survivors' ability to perceive humor may be impaired — cognition becomes more concrete and innuendo or concepts of humor may be entirely missed. Also, because of lack of self-confidence, survivors may be more self-conscious that we might be the butt of jokes — may be more sensitive to people laughing at rather than with us. Now's a good time to watch some comedies, read comic books, and attend improv classes!

What's the effect of your pre-injury personality?
While your previous personality influenced your responses, your injury exaggerated or revealed earlier traits. Some strong characteristics become stronger and others that were hidden are revealed — with both positive and negative results. This means that assertiveness may become aggression, agreeableness may change into passivity, determination into perseveration, a laid-back attitude into indifference, etc.

Risk-taking.
We TBI survivors typically took risks prior to the injury. It is likely that the same risk-taking personality traits will continue, unless/until insight, therapy, or medications intervene to affect them. And now, after the damage sustained, many of us are even less inhibited than before our injuries!

What is the predictable response of a risk taker who seems unable to do anything, let alone take risks? The behavior may surface in other potentially self-injurious ways: not complying with doctors' orders, like "forgetting" to take medications. If you are ambulatory, you may drive without a license, speed, drink and drive, or any number of other actions to take safety shortcuts, like not wearing a helmet or seat belt.

Addictive temperament.
My search for studies and observation of behaviors support my theory: *I have a feeling that we just might be addiction-prone. What do you think?*

Consider that addiction can be positive or negative. If you adopt a healthy addiction like physical fitness, it is positive. Using alcohol to excess or drugs or nicotine is counterproductive to your efforts to eat healthily and exercise. A helpful strategy is to ask yourself, "Do I want this or do I want to be fit?"

Substance Use and Abuse

Did you drink, drive, crash, and burn? You're not alone. For those survivors who didn't kill themselves outright, research shows that more than 60% of traumatic brain injuries involved the use of alcohol or other drugs. Here's the breakdown: 63% of falls, 66% of moving-vehicle accidents, and 71% of assaults were drug-related (Corrigan et al., 1995).

And between 38% and 50% of all survivors who made it to the emergency room were drunk (Kreutzer et al., 1996). Figures are not available for dead drunks, but severity of injury and pre-injury

> No one can make you feel inferior without your consent.
> — Eleanor Roosevelt

alcohol/drug patterns show it's not a pretty picture — survivors with a history of substance abuse suffered more severe injuries (Bigler et al., 1996). Survivors who abuse substances also don't return to productive activity and are less satisfied with life (Corrigan et al., 1997).

How does use differ from abuse and dependence?
They are different.

Use. Using mood-altering substances is considered "normal" and "acceptable" in many parts of our society. Consider the stimulation from caffeine or the relaxation of social drinking or the use of prescription drugs for relief of tension, pain, or insomnia. Substances can seem to enhance our lives.

Abuse. When use becomes abuse, drugs and alcohol lead to bad behavior. Substance abusers cannot control their use of alcohol or other drugs and regularly become intoxicated — whether on a daily, weekend, or binge basis — and often require the drug to function. Attempts to stop using are met with failure.

Dependence. Add to all the preceding symptoms a high tolerance (increasing amounts are required to achieve the desired effects) and a physical craving for the substance, be it alcohol, narcotics, amphetamines, or other drugs — then obtaining and using the drug of choice becomes the focus of life. If it is unavailable, addicts develop withdrawal symptoms within four to six hours that can last seven to ten days in the case of opiates. Some long-term addicts even lie awake and crave the drug for months!

Nicotine

Sorry, smokers! Nicotine's a chemical to avoid. Pre-injury, it was harmful — now it is even more so. Do your brain and other organs need the optimal amount of healthy blood to deliver nutrients — or not? Besides, how many people like to "kiss an ashtray" or be around someone who reeks of cigarette smoke? And consider the cost of those "butts" these days.

Don't blame yourself if you're addicted. According to recent research (Mameli-Engvall et al., 2006), your brain's reward systems are affected by the pleasurable effects of nicotine. But nicotine addiction can be treated!

How are smoking addictions treated?

Quitting is easier today than ever before! Smokers now do not have to go cold turkey or do it alone — or deprive themselves of pleasure. Western medicine offers numerous treatments for smoking addictions, including two pills and five different ways to receive nicotine and gradually decrease use — gum, inhaler, lozenge, patch, or nasal spray. Acupuncture treatments, as discussed in Chapter 8, also boast a high success rate.

Personal experience. Okay, I confess — I'm an ex-smoker. Because I smoked to relax, I promised myself that as soon as I reached the placid

Pacific, I'd quit. It wasn't exactly that fast, as smokers and ex-smokers understand, but to reduce a daily half-pack habit doesn't take very long. How did I quit? First I stashed emergency cigarettes next to my bed, in the car, and in the refrigerator — to remove the panic of deprivation. Then I followed two rules: I smoked only after running at low tide on the beach. If the tide didn't go out until late in the day, I waited until then. If a craving struck, I chewed on a piece of gum or something else, such as licorice, or engaged in a physical activity that used my hands. It's tough to ride a bicycle and smoke at the same time.

With these restrictions, quitting was relatively easy. I remember my last cigarette: I'd just finished a run and was warming down with a walk. As I lit up, I realized how silly I looked smoking a cigarette and wearing running attire. That was it.

Alcohol

Drinking patterns.
While it's not a surprise that guys drink more than gals, it's disturbing that survivors drink more than our non-injured peers. Forty-seven percent of male survivors consume moderate-to-heavy amounts of alcohol, in contrast to 38% of non-injured males. And 33% of female survivors report moderate-to-heavy consumption, compared to 17% of non-injured females (Corrigan, et al., 1995).

How does alcohol affect the brain?
By influencing neurotransmitters like dopamine and serotonin, alcohol produces a sense of well being and euphoria. *Are you familiar with this feeling?* Alcohol interferes with new brain cell growth and also impedes the brain's reorganization process after injury (UW, 1998).

Similar to the sedating and intoxicating properties of barbiturates and benzodiazepines like Valium, alcohol's net effect is to depress activity in the brain. Used medically, brain depressants can relieve anxiety and promote sleep. Small doses lead to calmness and relaxed muscles, while slightly larger amounts can cause poor judgment, slurred speech, staggering gait, and slow, uncertain reflexes.

Why is alcohol more damaging after TBI?
Studies of alcohol use after TBI find that cognitive, emotional, motor, and behavior performance deteriorate in those who use even "safe" amounts of alcohol and any previous impairments in these areas worsen (Corrigan et al., 1995; UW, 1998).

Although experts don't know all the reasons for the poor outcomes, theories point to alcohol's interference with neuronal sprouting. This interference results in rewiring connections that are haphazard and/or incorrectly linked. Spontaneous healing is also disrupted. Also, studies of brain tissues of alcoholics show that large quantities of alcohol cause neurological damage on their own — shrinking your brain! *Do we need this?!*

It is well known that drunkenness mimics brain injury, impairing attention, memory, judgment, and balance. What may not be known is that these impairments can last six weeks or more after stopping drinking, and permanently affect the brain of heavy drinkers (more than 10 drinks a day) or those over 40, according to Charles Bombardier at the University of Washington (1998). *So don't drink to get drunk anymore!*

Problems with alcohol use for survivors.
Here is a summary (Corrigan et al., 1995; UW, 1998; RTC, 2000) of the problems caused by alcohol:
- Alcohol disrupts healing and slows recovery.
- Alcohol interferes with psychoactive medications.
- Alcohol interferes with neuronal sprouting.
- Alcohol increases the risk of repeat injury and seizures.
- Alcohol increases the frequency of aggressive and/or anti-social behaviors.
- Alcohol worsens injury-related impairments — cognitive, motor, emotional, and behavioral — which then compromise vocational, academic, and psychological outcomes.

Marijuana

Although widely accepted and used by more than half of us survivors pre-injury, the use of "weed" after injury has not been studied yet. However, it is known to affect nearly all organ systems in our bodies, ranging from the central nervous system to the cardiovascular, endocrine, respiratory/pulmonary, and immune systems. Continued use can only further damage our injured brains. *As if we need to do that!*

As with every other action we take, health effects are determined by the age when use began as well as how often and how long someone uses. These are the known health hazards and effects of using marijuana (Khalsa et al., 2002; US Congress OTA, 1993):

Brain: cognitive.
For several days after use, marijuana impairs short-term memory, concentration, judgment, information processing, perception, and fine motor skills, thus increasing the risk of accidents (Corrigan et al., 1995). Driving skills are impaired for four to six hours after smoking one joint.

Brain: emotional/behavioral.
Marijuana causes chronic anxiety, depression, increased paranoia, and lifestyle changes such as apathy and concentration difficulties, which lead to declines in school and work performance and diminished abilities to carry out life plans in general.

Cardiovascular/respiratory system.
Marijuana significantly reduces lung function — more so than smoking tobacco, causes immediate increase in heartbeat and blood pressure, and leads to chronic cough and emphysema.

Cancer link.
Lung abnormalities suggestive of precancerous lesions have been found in marijuana users, as well as a risk of developing head, neck, and mouth cancer. There are even more carcinogens in marijuana than in tobacco cigarettes.

Immune system.
Marijuana impairs immune function, leading to increased vulnerability to infections.

Methamphetamine

This highly addictive central nervous system stimulant — also called "speed," "meth," or "crystal meth" — significantly changes how the brain functions, alters the dopamine system, reduces motor speed, and impairs verbal learning.

An intense rush that lasts only a few minutes follows smoking or injecting meth. Snorting produces effects within three to five minutes, while effects from oral ingestion take 15 to 20 minutes. Although the pleasurable effects disappear before the drug concentration in the blood falls significantly, users try to maintain the high by taking more of the drug, resulting in a binge-and-crash pattern (NIDA, 2006; NIDA, 2007). *Doesn't that sound like fun? — Not!*

Significantly, high doses of meth damage nerve cell endings, limiting regrowth. Studies also show severe structural and functional changes in areas of the brain associated with emotion and memory. Risks also increase for contracting HIV/AIDS, hepatitis B, and hepatitis C. Meth can also cause strokes (NIDA, 2006; NIDA, 2007).

If meth is ingested during pregnancy, risks include increased rates of premature delivery, fetal growth retardation, and birth defects in the heart and brain (NIDA, 2006).

Long-term effects of meth include paranoia, aggressiveness, convulsions, extreme and dangerous weight loss, memory loss, visual and auditory hallucinations, and severe dental problems.

Importantly, while some of the effects of chronic meth abuse appear to be at least partially reversible, function in some areas of the brain did not recover, even after two years of abstinence (NIDA, 2006).

Cocaine

Another stimulant of the central nervous system, cocaine causes chemical changes in the brain that lead to intense craving for more of the drug. As a stimulant, it provides a very temporary illusion of inexhaustible energy and power. The duration of the high depends upon how it's ingested. A snorting high may last 15 to 30 minutes, while a smoking high may last five to ten minutes. Increased use can reduce the duration of the high (NIDA, 2006). Other dose-related wide-ranging effects may include:

Brain: cognitive.
Cocaine causes confusion, impaired thinking, and incoherent talking. Cocaine-related blood pressure increases cause headaches and may rupture blood vessels in the brain, causing strokes and seizures (NIDA, 2004).

Brain: emotional/behavioral.
Cocaine damages brain cells that help produce pleasurable feelings, leading to depression. Hallucinations, restlessness, and anxiety are common, followed by deep depression. Other effects of cocaine include violent, erratic, paranoid behavior. Heavy cocaine users may experience fundamental personality changes, such as partial or total breaks with reality (Little et al., 2003; NIDA, 2003; NIDA, 2006).

Cardiovascular/respiratory system.
Cocaine increases blood pressure, heart rate, breathing rate, and body temperature. Cocaine can cause chest pain, cardiac arrhythmias, heart attacks, and strokes, as well as death from respiratory arrest. Regular cocaine snorting can lead to a chronically inflamed runny nose, nosebleeds, and loss of your sense of smell (Zickler, 2003). The cartilage structure of the nose can be destroyed by cocaine — *your nose can rot!*

Nervous and digestive systems.
Cocaine can cause dizziness, abdominal pain, nausea, tingling of hands and feet, and decreased appetite, which can lead to malnutrition.

Reproductive system/childbirth.
Cocaine can cause miscarriage, still birth, and premature labor or delivery. Exposure to cocaine in the womb can lead to many problems for babies: irritability, unresponsiveness to nursing and cuddling, permanent cognitive deficits, and an increased risk for seizures. Nursing babies who ingest cocaine in breast milk are prone to some of the same heart and brain problems as adults (Harvey 2004; NIDA, 2006).

Immune system.
Cocaine impairs your body's defense system for at least four hours, decreasing your ability to fight off infections (Zickler, 2004) and increasing your risk of contracting HIV and viral hepatitis (NIDA, 2004).

Patterns of use.
Typical patterns of use are near daily (chronic) and episodic (on weekends or at parties). Doses usually increase over time and binges are common. Binges terminate when either the user collapses or the cocaine supply runs out. A two-day crash period of recuperation generally follows the binge. *Doesn't this sound inviting?!*

Drug Combinations

As fun as it might sound, combining medications such as sedative-hypnotics with alcohol creates a potentially dangerous interaction — more toxic than either drug alone. The most common two-drug combination that leads to death is cocaine plus alcohol (NIA, 2004). Even after four weeks of abstinence from combined drugs, decreased cognitive functioning was apparent (Bolla et al., 2000). Combining drugs multiplies the effects of slowing down body functions and greatly increases the risk of death from overdose — whether accidental or not. *In this case, one plus one can equal zero!*

Survivor Substance Use and Abuse

We survivors partake of mind-altering substances for the same reasons non-injured folks do — to feel better! Depending on the substance, we can choose our emotion — peace, escape, relaxation, or excitement.

Why do we do this? Are survivors so injured — physically or psychologically — that we see no other alternatives? Is it mental — are we so weak-willed that we cannot stop ourselves? Is it emotional — are we so pleasure-driven that the "buzz" is worth the hang time? Is there a biochemical connection? And — is there any hope of change?

Genetic Factors and Chemical Connection

Genetic factors.

Yep, we can blame Mom and Dad for our use patterns. Results from both animal and human studies reveal that heredity influences use, misuse, and dependence on alcohol and other drugs. In fact, interviews of twins in Norway — where drug use is low — found that genetic factors play an important role in drug use (Kendler et al., 2006). This finding supported previous studies in the United States and Australia — where drug use is far higher. Additionally, a gene that alters the brain dopamine system contributes not only to alcohol abuse, but also to other eating and behavior disorders.

Alcohol impacts several *neurotransmitter* systems, especially dopamine and serotonin, that which are involved in the reward/reinforcement system in your brain. Research found lower levels of serotonin in alcoholics than non-alcoholics, a deficit of serotonin in alcohol-preferring rats, and that increasing serotonin levels in animals reduced voluntary alcohol intake (US Congress, OTA, 1993).

How can we blame Mom and Dad if we choose to drink too much? Abnormalities in the brain's serotonin system seem to play an important role in the brain's processes behind alcohol abuse. Low serotonin levels may contribute to the intoxicating effects and influence development of tolerance. Serotonin also affects alcohol consumption and its rewarding effects (Lovinger, 1999). Both dopamine and serotonin decrease during alcohol withdrawal, which illuminates the difficulties of quitting (Koob, 2006).

What exactly is inherited: biochemical, behavioral, or cultural traits? All three! Genetic differences have been found both in the intracellular mechanisms that control activity in some of the neurons in the brain reward system and in the number of neurons and receptors that contain dopamine in certain brain areas. Dopamine is the key neurotransmitter in cocaine's actions and the serotonin system regulates the activity of the dopamine system (US Congress, OTA, 1993).

Biochemical: the serotonin connection

Like a symphony conductor, the serotonin system balances and controls the effects of other neurotransmitters (the musical instruments), and regulates when or if they play. As the most common single neurotransmitter, serotonin directs the other neurotransmitters to coordinate a broad range of basic functions including the sleep/wake cycle, moods, appetite, motivation, and patterns of sensory and motor activity. At least fourteen different receptor subtypes are unlocked by the gatekeeper — serotonin.

Serotonin flicks the switch between alertness and asleep — the more active the serotonin system, the more alert the person. Serotonin causes the *metabolism* (breakdown) of *melatonin* during the night. The amount of *melatonin* regulates the sleep/wake cycle. When you awaken in the morning, light enters your retinas at the back of your eyes, melatonin production stops, and serotonin activity begins. Just as serotonin prompts us to move, physical activity also appears to regulate serotonin!

How the system operates plays a major role in how we feel. Fluctuations in our serotonin levels can determine if we're sad, glad, mad — or even bad! (Some violence disorders are related to deficient levels, too). Abnormalities in our brain's serotonin system play an important role in the brain processes behind addiction (Lovinger, 1999).

Importance to survivors.

If we haphazardly and unknowingly self-medicate our low serotonin levels, we interfere with rewiring our brains! Instead, consult an MD knowledgeable about substance abuse. A measured and constant dose of medication from the *SSRI* (selective serotonin-reuptake inhibitor) family can raise low serotonin levels. Also, try acupuncture. Acupuncture treatments also raise serotonin levels — which is why acupuncture is so effective with addictions!

Behavioral: What traits might be inherited?

While we know that alcoholism is quite rare in some cultures, most notably Asian, we may not understand the chemical connection. With two ineffective enzymes that metabolize (break down) alcohol in the body, even when Asians drink a small amount, it results in an obvious flushing of the face. If drinking continues, it may lead to nausea, dizziness, palpitations, and faintness. So, instead of a positive and reinforcing experience, drinking can provide a very negative experience for people of Asian heritage, which serves to prevent alcohol consumption, abuse, and dependence. This adverse reaction is common in 30 to 50 percent of the Asian people in Japan and Taiwan.

Studies of sons of alcoholics suggest the inherited risk of substance abuse also affects behavior. The studies found differences that affect temperament, learning styles, and the abilities and capacity to control behavior.

What determines the amount of impact of any substance? The particular *brain reward system* that is inherited (Mameli-Engvall et al., 2006; Koob, 2006; US Congress, OTA, 1993).

What is the brain reward system?
Reward reinforces behavior. Our brains are naturally wired to reward essential survival activities such as eating and drinking — but even without a survival goal, if the structures that are involved in the brain reward system are stimulated, pleasure alone is self-reinforcing. In other words, pleasure rules!

Studies have shown that animals will endure pain and even do without food and drink just to receive electrical stimulation to the reward system, explaining how drug-seeking behavior can rule addicts' lives.

Of the various brain structures that comprise this system, the key one is a neuronal pathway that connects structures in the middle part of your brain to those in the very front of your brain, in the prefrontal cortex. This part is often injured and is associated with control of emotion and behavior. *Do you see the connection?*

Is treatment for addictions successful?
Yes! And, now that you know that your brain reward system plays a central role in substance abuse, seek medical professionals who will treat your chemical imbalance as well as counsel you. For the best, and least frustrating, support, seek programs that offer a combined approach to TBI and substance abuse prevention. It also helps to find a mentor with a brain injury who currently attends a community-based program, such as

AA or NA. That person can help you understand the specific challenges of brain injury and help you make the program work.

Cognitive-behavioral therapy and contingency management.
These are effective individual and group treatments for all substance use and the best ones for methamphetamine addiction. Cognitive-behavioral therapy helps clients analyze why and when they use and how to cope better with problems. The comprehensive "matrix model" includes family education and 12-Step support. Contingency management provides incentives in exchange for engaging in treatment.

Self-help programs.
These include twelve-step approaches, such as Alcoholics (AA), Narcotics (NA), and Cocaine Anonymous (CA) as well as Rational Recovery and Moderation Management for alcohol problems. These approaches focus on developing personal responsibility within the context of peer support.

Residential treatment programs.
These can teach users how to live in society again and offer vocational rehab and other supportive services. Some, like Therapeutic Community (TC), involve stays for 6 to 12 months.

Medication treatment.
Prescription medications for depression or anxiety can help, especially when beginning a program. Medication such as Acamprosate (Campral) can reset the neurochemical system to maintain abstinence by reducing craving and relapse drinking (To, 2006). Others work in different ways. Different medications may be combined. Discuss options with your doctor.

Community-based programs.
The most effective ones include health, financial, social, and vocational areas. If treatment begins within three months of injury, survivors are more likely to both maintain abstinence and be productive.

In addition to significantly less alcohol consumed and/or less frequent use three to four years post-injury, nearly 60% of the participants were also employed, in school or training, or volunteering post-treatment, as opposed to nearly 70% either not working or not in school prior to treatment (Corrigan et al., 1996).

Emotional Issues

Recovery from a broken brain is a pain! Here are some of our challenges:

> Happiness is a thing to be practiced, like the violin.
> — John Lubbock

Failure

How often do you feel like you can't do something — or anything? Remember, physical damage causes this difficulty — not that you're not trying. "Perhaps you're doing something like you did it pre-injury and need to adapt to a different way" (C. Baser, 1997). Work hard in therapy to find new methods!

Control and Responsibility

Do you feel powerless over your body and your mind? — even over your very being? To feel some sense of control, act like you want it — don't ask others to perform tasks that you can do. The more you do, the more you'll be able to do — the less you do, the less you'll be able to do!

Clamor Control: The Nightmare of Noise

Shreeeeeeeeeeeeeeeek. Clattttttttter. The sudden shriek of a train horn that blasts for two hundred yards or the mile-long rumble and clatter of a freight train may be only minor, short-lived annoyances for non-injured folks. For us survivors, they can be major, ear-splitting disruptions.

Personal experience. As we prepared for a bike ride after a restful night and a peaceful breakfast at her home in the country, it happened. There was no warning, just that awful screaming blower noise that provides its own version of surround sound. I tried to continue getting ready, pumping air into the tires, inserting the filled water bottles into the cages. I was shaking so badly that I dropped one of the bottles, cursed, and then lost control entirely, yelling and sobbing, rolling around on the concrete driveway. My friend guided me inside. The sobs started again. She comforted me like a baby as I lay on the floor. (I did remember to ground myself.) Later, Christine advised me: "Don't try to continue what you are doing. Go away or otherwise protect yourself from the noise. Do not try to ignore it and continue what you're doing."

Sources of distress.
Any loud, unpredictable, or sudden noise can make us feel overwhelmed!

What to do.
Prepare and protect! To feel a sense of control, avoid known causes of distress. For unavoidable irritants:

- Insulate your ears. Try headphones or surround yourself with the white noise of an electric fan, soothing sounds like moving water, or relaxing music.
- Fight back! Use your hair dryer or vacuum or some other loud appliance that you can control.
- Practice a ritual, like meditation, yoga, or tai chi.
- Structure daily activities so you feel some control.
- Consider ways to cope before you blow your circuits — saving not only yourself, but also your family and friends.
- Accept that noise bothers you and that you need to compensate or suffer the consequences.

Swearing

Frequent swearing is another post-injury behavior that plagues us. Even if we rarely or never swore before the injury, now we may curse almost involuntarily as well as an in anger. Here are some solutions:

- Reduce emotional stressors to stay peaceful.
- Use other words. Foreign curse-words may work — if no one near you speaks that language!
- Substitute a less offensive word, like "darn."
- Create a new word with harsh "k" or "t" sounds.
- Do something else when you feel like swearing.

SSSSSSStuttering

After injury, stuttering, stammering, and other language problems (both in talking and listening) are common. These are worsened by emotional stress. Some solutions:

- Sing! Because singing bypasses the speech-specific language center, stuttering doesn't occur, regardless of stress.
- Practice maintaining a calm spirit by playing relaxing music and performing meditative exercises like yoga, tai chi, etc.

Outbursts

Try to head them off before they occur! List constructive ways to defuse and redirect your anger. Be alert to the warning signs of an outburst. Because many of us aren't able to tell when we're about to explode, ask a loved one to warn you. *Some of us are a bit slow in this area. It took me about fifteen years to know that an eruption was imminent.*

Specific Helpful Behaviors

Let's look at some specific behaviors that will help you get through these emotional issues sooner.

Exercise.
The more vigorous the better — exercise is one of the best responses to anger. Anything that uses a lot of mental or physical energy can diminish built-up rage. Exercise also helps to overcome and reduce depression. Sustained movement increases energy, improves self-esteem, and lessens tension and fatigue. TBI exercisers not only experience less depression, but also fewer cognitive problems (RTC, 1999).

Find and use verbal support.
Because we survivors often become more externally motivated after the injury, due to diminished self-trust, a vote of confidence by a significant person is powerful.

Personal experience. One of DJ's most helpful statements went something like this: "Soon you'll find that a part of each day won't be so awful. Then, a bigger part, which will progress to a whole day that is mostly good. Soon, there will be several days in the week that are more good than bad. Eventually, you will experience more joy than sadness in entire weeks." Why did this work? Because I believed DJ — he'd been right at other times. Because he said it would happen, it did happen, like a self-fulfilling prophecy. It provided hope and fuel for my very tenuous hold on life. Now most of my days are mostly happy.

Recall motivational words from respected sources.

Personal experience. My father, a former coach, encouraged me: "Do one more than you think you can, Honey." This worked because it placed responsibility on me to accomplish my goals, and it showed he thought I could do one more, which inspired me to actually do two more!

Listen to motivational audio or videotapes.
Select and use tapes that speak most directly to you!

Display uplifting visual reminders.
Post a sign on your wall that says, "You're a winner!" or another phrase that reminds you that you can make it.

Consider keeping a pet.
Not only do pets provide silent, unconditional love, they often sense what to do. Caring for a pet offers diversion and a sense of control over something. *Fish are easy!*

Make some choices/decisions that affect you and others.
Deciding what and when to eat or when and if to go somewhere lets you practice being in control of what happens to you.

Seek community enrichment resources.
Seek your own answers. We live in the information age — use it and enjoy it!

Create!
Use your senses to both vent and invent. Write, draw, work with clay, paint, or other media; sing or play a musical instrument.

Personal experience. My quick wit was a former personality trademark that I cherished — and fondly remember. Losing that fun part of my personality lessened my overall joy. So, ever the student, I enrolled in improv comedy classes with a couple of my nuttier friends. What happened? I couldn't remember what I was supposed to do! Did this turn into yet another example of failure? No, because I played the dummy and moved my hands to my friend's talking. What did I learn? Three things: if there is an activity that requires memory, cue cards are essential; evening hours after 8 PM generally are a poor time for learning, even after a nap; and frequent laughter helps recovery!

Do relaxing activities.
Listen to music, read, or meditate.

Do "create-to-destroy" activities.
Release angry and sad feelings through burning, shredding, cutting, or burying items that are specifically designed to be destroyed. Pictures, written notes, letters, drawings, or crafted art objects can all be used (Baser, 1997).

Summary

Yes, you can! You can rewire successfully. You can eventually find a way through, over, under, or around the circuit breakers as you seek balance — if you stay connected to God and others. "Keep knocking on doors!"

Personal experience. Encountering — and overcoming — steep climbs on a recent bicycle ride reminded me of the recovery journey. I didn't know the exact route when I started — only that if I

> Happiness is a thing to be practiced, like the violin.
> — John Lubbock

wanted to ride with my triathlon club I needed to be able to do "the lake loop." I felt prepared and energetic that day, so decided to ride past my usual turn-around and explore. After a couple of difficult ascents, I thought, "Oh, this isn't so bad — I can do this!" When the climbs continued I looked harder for the "loop" around the lake. Then when I saw a sign indicating that the next turn was 17 miles away, I thought,

"Oh! It can't be any worse than what you've ridden, so let's keep going."
When another very steep rise loomed ahead I began to doubt my
decision. But the closer I came to the hill, the flatter it seemed! I
chuckled as I realized how similar this bike ride was to the ups and
downs of the recovery journey and how, if we just keep going, the road
flattens out. Just do it!

Here is a list of ideas to help you emotionally rewire:
- Avoid known causes of distress.
- Ask, what do I need to be calm?
- Ask, who can help me?
- Practice a ritual like meditation, yoga, or tai chi.
- Recall motivational words from respected sources.
- Structure daily activities to feel some control.
- Consider ways to cope before you blow your circuits.
- Find and use verbal support.
- Remember that the physical damage causes you to fail at something — not that you're not trying.
- Use motivational tapes (audio or video).
- Display uplifting reminders. ("You're a winner!")
- Consider keeping a pet. *Fish are easy!*
- Seek community enrichment resources and use them!
- Get active — do anything that brings you joy!
- Don't use/abuse substances (cigarettes, alcohol/drugs).
- Realize that grieving and accepting your loss may take many years.
- Use the SAFER method (Stop, Assess, Fix, Examine, Retry).
- Believe that you are okay — just different from what you were.
- Know that you can be better — but only if you work at it!

7

Body-Mind Rewiring: Healing with Conventional Medicine

Remember to cure the patient as well as the disease.

— Dr. Alvin Barach

"Help! I'm fried! Where are those circuits and which wire goes where?"

Sometimes it seems we're connected and spliced to every imaginable power source. Other times we lack wires, plugs, links, and even current. Perhaps drained, not charged by all the power surges over time, we may feel even weaker with each new "cure." Sometimes we don't know how we feel — except frustrated — with dangling wires and interrupted current to prove it.

Our minds, bodies, and spirits must work together and with medicine and its providers — however we define it and whoever practices it. Most certainly, we must not give our power away — to anyone. Doctors are instruments of healing we have chosen to assist us to regain our own health. To prevent relinquishing too much power to others, I propose that whatever treatments you choose make sense to you. Not that it always has to make intellectual sense, but that it makes sense to your gut, which was not damaged and speaks clearly if you choose to listen to it.

To rewire, we need to know which treatment wires to plug in and who and what can help us. And, if you try a treatment and it doesn't work, try something else. Conventional medicine topics include:

- Psychiatric care and medications.
- Psychological care: traits of helpful and non-helpful therapists.
- Neuropsychological care.
- Psychological talk-therapy interventions, EMDR, and neurofeedback.
- Vision and inner-ear therapy.
- Physical therapy, including therapeutic horseback riding.
- Recreational therapy, including animal-assisted therapy.
- Expressive arts therapies: art, music, drama, dance/movement.
- Therapeutic devices: light boxes and electrical stimulation units.
- Self-advocacy with health professionals.

Psychiatric Care and Medications

Medications can help with some of the problems caused by a head injury. Let's look at some of the places you should think about taking medications.

Depression.

"I don't need a shrink and drugs. I'll be fine — I'm just tired. Just leave me alone so I can sleep!"

> Even if you are on the right track, you will get run over if you just sit there.
> — Will Rogers

Is this really what you want?

"Well, maybe not, but what can I do about it?"

Get help — unless you want to keep feeling that way. After brain injury, irritability and fatigue are common and many of us feel depressed. In fact, researchers estimate from 27% to 59% of all survivors experience an injury-induced depression (Seel et al., 2003; Moldover et al., 2004). But it can be treated so you feel better!

"Depressed — who, me?"

Yep. If you experience five or more of the following symptoms, lasting two weeks or more and not due to any other physical condition, substance, or medication, get help!

- Persistently depressed, sad, anxious, or empty.
- Worthless, helpless, or very guilty.
- Hopeless and pessimistic about the future.
- Lack of interest and pleasure in your usual activities.
- Low or no energy; chronic fatigue.
- Poor memory; difficulty making decisions or concentrating.
- Irritable, restless, or agitated.
- Sleep disturbances: either difficulty falling asleep, staying asleep, or sleeping too much.
- Loss of appetite and interest in food or overeating/weight gain.
- Frequent thoughts of death or suicidal thoughts or actions.

Basically, if you're depressed, you hate life and everything about it, with no energy or desire to do anything about this feeling and no hope that it will change. It's the Three-P Plight: "The feeling is permanent, pervasive, and personal" (Baser, 1998). Even if you experience fewer than five symptoms, tell your doctor, loved ones — anyone. Just get help!

Personal experience. *By 1990 I was both anti-drug and anti-MDs, so I never thought I'd ask a doctor for a prescription. But as my therapist, Christine, and I talked about my deep depression and the effectiveness of new drugs, she told me about someone who worked with survivors and was an expert on medications, but didn't push pills. Imagine my surprise when the doctor she recommended, Daniel Gardner, was the author of an article in the* Brain Injury Press *that had both surprised and impressed me! Here was a physician who was honest about his own previous reluctance to prescribe drugs, so I had to give him a try!*

After so many drugged-out months in the '70s, however, I was very reluctant to voluntarily take this path again. Dr. Gardner understood and assured me that the new medications would not leave me in a stupor, but would balance my serotonin levels so my brain would work and I would feel better. He suggested that we start at a very low dose, see how it worked, and adjust it when necessary. I stayed on this regimen for ten years until I switched to a Cranial Electrical Stimulator (CES) device.

Because Dr. Gardner trusted me to follow the rules, I regulated my own Prozac level from 1.5 mg to 20 mg, depending upon how I assessed my mood. If anyone else was brave enough to suggest that I might need an increase, I thought about it. Because we both believed in body-speak, this approach worked.

Medication use: what do I need to understand about treatment?
Obviously, the benefits should outweigh the risks. For example, is it possible that the medication could worsen your depression or cause other cognitive and physical problems? After deciding to include medication as part of a treatment plan, do/consider the following:

- Use the lowest effective dose to minimize side effects.
- Monitor symptoms, both positive and negative.
- Report any side effects, then discuss options: changing dose, changing or adding medication. Undergo blood tests as recommended by your doctor.
- Know that several factors affect absorption levels, including: weather, food and beverage intake, and interactions with other prescription and over-the-counter medications.
- Give the medication time to work. It may take four to eight weeks, depending on the type.
- Accept and understand the role of medication in general and the actions of the particular medications prescribed (Gardner, 1992, 2007).

Why would I want to use medications?
So you can rule yourself, rather than your symptoms or some alien ruling you. The goal of medications is to correct the balance of your neurotransmitters so you can heal yourself. When your brain works properly, you can productively use your psychotherapy sessions so they become action-oriented instead of complaint-oriented. Basically, taking medications is like wearing a cast to allow a broken bone to heal — the real work begins after the cast stabilizes the bone.

What are some mistaken ideas about using medications?
It's both common and dangerous to think that the drugs will fix everything that's wrong so you can veg out in front of the TV. It's also a mistake to consider medications unnatural. Drugs are remedies that may be natural or manufactured. Anything we ingest can be considered a drug.

Don't pay attention to people who criticize you for being weak and using "a crutch." How smart is it to not use a crutch to help your body repair itself? *"See how strong I am! I don't need a crutch for my broken leg — I'll just limp the rest of my life."* The biggest factor in recovery is not pills, but how motivated you are. How badly do you want to rewire?

> What do you want — a nickel today or a quarter tomorrow?
> — Dale Johnson (DJ)

Personal experience. Thanks to good "shrinks," my overheard suicide-or-state-hospital prediction did not come to pass between my accident in 1976 and today despite some of my efforts — God wasn't finished with me yet! After a lot of banging on doors (and a few other things), I eventually found the professional connections that worked for me. I remain plugged in to all of them, linked either by memory or by contact. Keep knocking on doors or desks — whatever works!

Psychological Care

From darkness to light. Anyone who's lived in the black hole of depression knows how that shock feels — the spark of life forged by a galvanized connection to the correct transformer. If the time is right and the plugs match — electricity!

> A merry heart doeth good like a medicine, but a downcast spirit drieth the bones.
> — Proverbs 17:22

Oh, the hope we feel when we connect with the right psychotherapist! The connection, whether short or long, turns on our power at the correct wattage and boosts output, without overloading our wires. It may be low or high voltage, but it's what we need.

Traits of the most helpful therapists.

- That I had brain damage was believed, with or without evidence.

> Absence of proof isn't proof of absence!
> — Nathan Zasler

- We connected. They liked me and showed me respect.
- If I was in bad shape and needed more time, our sessions were extended or extra meetings were scheduled.
- In emergencies, by following our rules I could call DJ at home or page Christine.
- They responded to emergency pages and any other calls.
- They were all highly intelligent and respected my abilities, too.
- They were honest, confronting, and loving — all at once!
- They trusted me and weren't alarmed by anything I did or said.
- They looked at me and responded rather than just taking notes.
- They used a non-conventional approach with a flexible structure.
- We agreed on treatment methods to use and the desired outcomes.
- They wanted to learn about me from significant people in my life.
- I found them through a physical ailment (ulcers), traumatic life event (rape, accidents), or the reliving of an awful event.
- They referred me to other people/places and suggested homework.
- The therapists were all within 10 years of my age.
- All relationships were long-term, usually two to five years.

Personal experience. *To use anger in more productive ways was one of my major therapeutic needs. Here's how star therapist DJ handled me:*

> Don't push the river; it flows by itself.
> — DJ

Me: (kicking the desk) "How many doors do I have to knock on?"

DJ: "As many as it takes; you might want to save your energy."

This interchange shows the wry — and not always gentle — humor that was so important for me. This tough, yet caring approach prodded me back to problem solving and away from the "poor me" whining that seems typical for many of us, regardless of our progress on our journey.

The therapists who were unhelpful or destructive also shared many traits. See the list in Chapter 7 of *Brain Injury Rewiring for Loved Ones.*

Neuropsychological Care

You will probably connect — at least short-term — with a specially trained psychologist called a neuropsychologist. These doctors determine how a brain injury impacts how we think, feel, and act. Then using their experience and results from tests, they help us and our families understand the changes, set realistic daily goals, and make short- and long-range plans.

Neuropsychologists can work their magic with us in talk therapy because they understand injury-caused deficits. Together we examine how what we think, feel, and do is affected by what is going on within us and around us — and how we can obtain and maintain balance. By empowering and encouraging us to move from a victim mentality to a proactive stance, they help us to learn how to adapt, compensate, and gradually accept the "new person with the same name."

Together, we explore strategies to deal with specific problems such as disturbed sleep or sensitivity to noise, as well as complex problems like depression, memory loss, fears, or anxieties. We also discuss "Who am I now and how do I get along with my family and friends?" and "What kind of work can I do and how do I find it?"

Some neuropsychologists are trained in cognitive therapy. This talk therapy helps us to redefine and revise negative thoughts and beliefs that cause us stress as well as bad behavior! For example, if someone doesn't acknowledge us, it doesn't necessarily mean they're ignoring us. Maybe they're preoccupied with something else or don't see us (Baser, 1998). *Cognitive override works for me — whenever I think to use it!*

There are so many therapies today that can help us! I hope that everyone will connect with at least one of the "hot wires" in this next section.

Eye Movement Desensitization and Reprocessing (EMDR)

We all know that trauma disrupts balance. What we may not know is how to restore it. We want harmony back — now! — before the trauma or post-traumatic stress disorder (PTSD) controls our life any longer.

Perhaps it's time for the magic of EMDR. This non-invasive psychotherapeutic technique uses your rapid eye movements (or sounds or taps) to permanently and rapidly restore lost harmony by freeing brain waves to once again move together on both sides of the brain. Relief may be felt after one session and typically in ten sessions or less (Robinson, 1992; Bennington, 1997).

EMDR recreates the body's natural way of reintegrating events — dreaming. Similar or identical to the involuntary rapid eye movement (REM) that occurs when we dream, these rhythmic eye movements allow the painful memory to be desensitized (Marsa, 2002).

When the rhythmic eye movements stimulate the processing system, it allows our memory to remember the event, but disables the negative emotions associated with it. EMDR works to correct abnormal brain processing and desynchronized brain waves, both caused by trauma's intensity. Lateral eye movements free the stuck effects of trauma to enable normal neuronal activity to resume, reintegrating the memory of the event, according to the developer of the technique, Francine Shapiro, PhD. (Weil, 1997).

Personal experience. EMDR works! See Chapter 7 in *Brain Injury Rewiring for Loved Ones* to read more about it.

Biofeedback

We'll talk about how practitioners of traditional Chinese medicine redirect body energy without the use of a machine in the next chapter. In the technology-happy West people often prefer to hook up with a device to train themselves to manipulate their brain activity.

Using lab procedures developed in the 1940s, the Western form of biofeedback enables people to control such supposedly involuntary functions as heart rate, blood pressure, muscle tension, and blood supply to the skin by using signals from their bodies (Miller, 2008; La Fazio, 1997).

How does biofeedback work? What conditions can it treat?

The biofeedback machine acts like a camera to show changes in muscle activity. Connected by sensors to a device that picks up electrical signals from your muscles, you see and hear your tension "fed back" to you with visual and auditory cues that are displayed on a computer monitor.

Muscles under stress contract and cause pain. You learn to associate sensations in your muscles with levels of tension that are reflected in the cues given by the machine. To slow down the flashing or beeping signals on the screen requires relaxing your tense muscles. With continued training, you can learn to relax your muscles at will, and thus alter your physiological responses, gradually doing it without the machine (La Fazio, 1997).

Biofeedback can treat any condition that is affected by stress. Importantly for survivors, it is effective with both tension and migraine headaches, as well as many other types of chronic pain and disorders of the digestive and respiratory systems.

Neurofeedback

Neurofeedback is noninvasive electronic biofeedback that uses an EEG machine to continuously measure the brain's activity. You receive information about incorrect brain waves from the computer through sound, sight, or touch. Because your brain receives this feedback at the time of each error, it knows what the problem is and can quickly correct itself, empowering you to heal yourself.

Neurofeedback helps symptoms to diminish, and the entire system is moved toward higher functioning and wellness within seven sessions, although at least forty sessions will be necessary for permanent benefits. As in all learning, practice makes perfect (Dupler, 1998).

Vision Therapy

Just as you look into someone's eyes to determine if they're telling the truth, your eyes also serve as the primary doorway to the world and a gauge of your total health.

If you find it difficult to maintain your balance and feel uncoordinated, your vision might be impaired. Survivors often experience blurry and double vision, as well as light sensitivity.

This optical damage may delay proper rehabilitation because professionals may mistake visual dysfunction for behavioral, psychiatric, and/or cognitive problems. We're not nuts — we just can't see!! Working with specialists could return full function. If not, you'll learn compensatory practices, such as how to use special prisms and mirrors, and/or modify the environment. *My favorite: fix the environment!*

Personal experience. Visual therapy at the Optometric Vision Development Center was so helpful to me! Dr. Claude Valenti's assistant Lenore lovingly coached me through a variety of drills, some of which were fun, others challenging, and still others boring — all of them part of my rewiring plan. Take-home devices, some of which I still use, encouraged me to practice, especially with lots of computer time.

Balance Disorders

Because most of us experience balance problems, it is likely that your injury produced an inner-ear disorder that affects your balance. Some of us feel dizzy or a false sense of motion, like spinning. Others may feel themselves falling, rising, and rocking.

For any balance difficulty, consult a specialist because the damage may be subtle and the symptoms vague, as is typical with brain injury. A brief exam by a generalist is not likely to find the cause of the seemingly minor damage, particularly if you are lying down. Correct detection and diagnosis often requires movement.

What kinds of therapy are used for balance disorders?

Although treatment methods depend upon the disorder, balance retraining is a typical approach, regardless of the source of the problem. For those of us with the common disorder known as Benign Paroxysmal Positioning Vertigo (BPPV), several positioning techniques are used to help us maintain our center of gravity. Gait retraining is also used (Gizzi, 1995; Shumway-Cook, 2003). Balance training works — give it a try!

Physical Therapy (PT)

Naturally, with my repeated use of the "practice, practice, practice" directive, it's no surprise that I cheer the vital role of physical activity. This section focuses on working with others to heal us. Work with them and *"Just do it!"* Then enjoy the benefits! You may not always enjoy the work, but you will always enjoy the results!

Why do I need PT and what will I do there?
Do you want greater independence? More fun? Or just to feel better? By now you know that if you increase physical strength, cardiovascular endurance, balance, and flexibility, you also improve your ability to function. This means greater confidence and independence, which leads to a more active social life — and who knows where they all may lead!

Even with paralysis and weakness, survivors can become more independent, feel better, and be more in control when we strengthen what remains and learn how to adapt for what is lost. How? Participate in a training program, first with a physical therapist, and then independently. Do you want to work with a robot? New robotic devices are available now to help you regain use of a damaged limb. See *Brain Injury Rewiring for Loved Ones*, Chapter 7, to learn more.

In PT you will become acquainted with your body again. After you warm up for a few minutes on an arm bike, leg bike, treadmill, or other piece of cardio equipment, your physical therapist will move your body to see what it can do compared to your last session. You will learn what to do to move better, stronger, and easier. With an individually designed program and under supervision, you will use various machines, exercise cords, balls, and fun — and not so fun! — equipment to achieve your goals.

More than just designers of tortuous exercise programs, physical therapists offer activities to fit any needs and use water and animal therapies to help us rewire. Dance and movement therapy are included in the Expressive Arts section of this chapter, so keep reading! They're all fun!

What kinds of goals can I set? How do I achieve them?
Whatever you choose! Standard goals include improving overall functioning, strength, endurance, balance, and flexibility. Goals may also include learning how to use adaptive devices.

To achieve your goals, "just do it!" with effort, will power, and perseverance! First, a therapist directs your exercise program, then you work on your own doing the same or similar exercises.

If you continue to work, you will continue to improve — it's that simple! I'm 30-plus years post-injury and getting better all the time. While it's a journey with many detours, rewiring continues if mind and body are challenged, just as with non-injured folks. It's fun for me because I often wonder, "How good can I get?" You can improve, too!

Personal experience. It's PT again for me after another detour! I recently learned that a surfing injury six years ago caused permanent nerve damage and paralysis to two of the four rotator cuff muscles in my dominant arm and shoulder. So that's why my swimming stroke and surf paddling is weak! What to do? The physical therapist will design a program to strengthen surrounding musculature and compensate for the muscles that no longer work. She will also monitor my form in the strengthening exercises so I can relearn how to use that arm without further injuring and causing pain to that shoulder. I still plan to make Team USA in triathlon — it'll just take longer, like maybe after I'm 65 years old. Never ever quit is my motto!

> The greatest danger for most of us is not that our aim is too high and we miss it, but that it is too low and we reach it.
> — Michelangelo

Aquatic therapy

A therapy pool provides buoyancy, resistance, warmth, stress relief, and a social environment — what more could we ask for! For those of us with balance difficulties, walking in water helps us develop better sensory awareness and it doesn't hurt when we fall! Different kinds of flotation devices add to the experience and make it more fun. Others in the pool also working to improve their condition makes it feel like a pool party!

Hippotherapy (therapeutic horseback riding)

Here's a therapy designed especially by and for survivors! Because a horse's gait is similar to a human's gait, it's natural to use a horse to treat people with movement disorders, right? Plus, it's fun!

During therapy, a rider is placed in different positions on the horse to take advantage of the horse's movement. The rider also performs various exercises and plays games while on horseback (NCEFT, 1997).

Recreational Therapy

Animal-assisted therapy (AAT)

They pay attention on demand, ease depression, give unconditional love and free physical therapy. They like a slow pace. They're blind to age, color, disability, and even body odor. Their needs are few. They're free or cheap. Huh? Who and where is this angel — in heaven?

> People make great companions for cats...all a cat has to do is purr and rub against their legs every now and then and they're content.
> — Morris, the Cat

These healers come in many sizes and shapes. Some weigh less than an ounce and some weigh more than a ton. They may have two legs or four. They may be furry or fuzzy, scaly, finned, or feathered. Without a voice, they speak to our souls.

Called "Angel Animals" by some, spiritual companions by others, pets help us heal and socialize — at our rate. Dogs can open doors — literally and figuratively — at home and in the community.

Physically, animals encourage us to exercise, reduce our blood pressure, and redirect our attention away from pain. Socially, we experience less boredom and more communication and recreation. Emotionally, we're less anxious and lonely (Voelker, 1995).

Speech-Language Therapy

These therapists can energize an entire circuit, as the following story witnesses. Some professionals, like San Diego's Joanne Hein, host monthly meetings where survivors exchange solutions to current rewiring problems. With no one else there, we have no choice but to communicate with each other!

Personal experience. *Finally! A proper response to my plaintive cry: "I won't be so upset all the time if my brain works!" Disgruntled, and* *either rowdy — who, me? — or in a drug-induced stupor, I bounced from one psychiatric ward to another for years, repeating my mantra "Fix my brain and I won't be crazy!" Picture Jack Nicholson in* One Flew over the Cuckoo's Nest!

At last, I was heard! My speech therapist, Eugenia Don, actually asked me what I wanted to achieve! Thanks to the speech-language program designed by her, my cognitive skills improved — and so did my emotional control (duh!), Does this show that patients often know what they need — just not where to find it? Twice a week for one year, I enjoyed our cognitive rehabilitation sessions. Eugenia even developed take-away notebooks that were so fun to do that I worked on vacations! May God bless you, Eugenia, wherever you are!

And, true to the "pass it on" directive, several others — both sick and well — benefited from the emotional lift of our sessions: Immediately after my high with Eugenia, I visited my dear friend from church, Lucille Carolyn Dare, who resided in one of the nearby convalescent homes. We, in turn, brought cheer to others in the home! And, because Eugenia empowered me, I could effectively advocate for Lucille, easing her life and reassuring her worried Texas relatives and local church friends who also cared for her. At last, I was a helper — a "wounded healer" — and not a helpee!

Occupational Therapy

Do you need to learn how to function one-handed in a two-handed world? Loving educators called OTRs, the acronym for Occupational Therapists Registered teach us ways to adapt our environment and everything in it to fit our needs.

Personal experience. Needing pain relief and support for a thumb injury a few years ago, I contacted a local OTR for help. If you ever wonder why you need a thumb, ask someone to splint yours and try to do anything! Beyond daily activities, I also need mine to write, bicycle, and lift weights, so my clever therapist constructed several splints for me to wear (day, night, and activity). And Leucadia Cyclery bike genius, Fred, devised different handlebar grips so I could ride safely without pressure on my sore thumb. The team approach came to the rescue again!

Expressive Arts

You rediscovered in Spiritual Rewiring how to tap your creative energy to heal body, mind, and spirit using the arts. When the nervous system changes from stressed and perhaps fearful to peaceful,

> He who sings frightens away his ills.
> — Miguel De Cervantes Saavedra

relaxed, and creative, different brain wave patterns are produced that increase learning, creativity, and dreaming. This section explores how specialists use the arts to help us deal with our injuries and help us heal.

Art therapy

The art we produce may symbolize our inner world, make talking easier, or just be a way to express our feelings.

Music therapy

As we know, music is almost magic: it calms and relaxes, eases pain, counters depression, and stimulates movement. Trained to know how certain types of music affect our behavior, music

> Music is the shorthand of emotion.
> — Leo Tolstoy

therapists devise activities to help us improve our physical, emotional, and social skills. We play instruments, sing, move, or just listen to music to speed our recovery.

Drama therapy

Another fun way to access feelings is by acting them out, with or without words — either through improvisational theater or scripted scenes. Some of us find it easier to show how we feel than talk about it or create a work of art that represents it.

Also termed "psychodrama," therapeutic theater offers a fresh and sometimes funny view of potentially painful thoughts, feelings, and past events under the watchful eye and direction of a skilled drama therapist. *Try it — it's safe and fun!*

Movement/dance therapy

Many of us fondly remember when we first moved in response to music or mimicked animals and their gestures. Capture the fun and joy of this again through movement therapy! In response to music, suggestions, scripts, or improvisational material, movement therapy challenges us to explore feelings in yet another way — and it is such fun to play!

> Use what talents you possess: the woods would be very silent if no birds sang there except those that sang best.
> — Henry Van Dyke

Personal Therapeutic Devices

Here are three that I find especially helpful: light boxes, cranial electrical stimulation, and nerve stimulation units.

Light Box

Thanks to technology, we can now ease depression in front of our own light box, balance our brain, and reduce pain with electrical impulses — without drugs or knives!

"Treat my depression with a light box? What a ridiculous idea!" Is it absurd if it works? Using light boxes to treat depression may seem outrageous, but not if we consider why light therapy works.

Our bodies need 30-120 minutes of natural sunlight or special artificial light every day for physical and emotional health. Light is vital for brain functioning, including balancing our circadian rhythm. Do you ever wonder why we're drowsy at night? Darkness kicks in the production of the natural hormone melatonin. Light stops this action.

Who's light deprived? What are the symptoms?

Millions of people need more light than they get, especially in the winter. Most of these live in northern climates, although anyone can be affected by loss of light.

Is your sleep disturbed? Are you anxious, sad, tired? Do you just want to be alone? Is your energy low? Do you experience trouble concentrating and being productive? Besides depression, inadequate light has been linked to these other health problems (*Health Confidential*, 1996; Tufts, 1994). See Chapter 7 in *Brain Injury Rewiring for Loved Ones* for more information.

Personal experience. I love my light box! Ever since 1990 I've happily used it all year round to read the newspaper while eating breakfast (about 30-60 minutes). After I was assaulted at the home of my client by a deranged former aide and then developed clinical depression, my psychiatrist suggested I use the light box twice a day, in the morning and at lunch as late as 2 PM. That new plan and an additional 300 mg of Neurontin worked — the depression gradually faded, helped by the summer sun!

Cranial Electrical Stimulation

Here is my other favorite anti-depression apparatus that I control, the CES unit.

"Use electricity to rewire my brain cells? Huh? This I've gotta hear!"

Using a palm-sized device powered by one 9V battery, you can stimulate your brain to relieve depression, anxiety, pain, insomnia — and even chemical addictions! (Klawansky et al., 1995).

How does a CES unit work? How do I use it?

CES quiets the mind and brings balance. Electrodes, located on a head set or on ear lobe clips or affixed behind the ears with gel, send a current that is felt as a mild and pleasant tingling sensation.

Time of use depends upon what condition you're treating. If you seek relief from insomnia and/or depression, 20-40 minutes daily for the first month is suggested, then as needed. Perhaps using it every other day will work, or even every three days. As soon as you begin to feel depressed again, resume use! For anxiety, stress, and/or pain, use as needed. If you feel burning, decrease the setting. If you don't feel anything, add moisture to the pads and/or reposition them. Replace or wash dirty pads and replace the battery when the power is low, indicated by a blinking red light.

Personal experience. I'm very happy with my CES unit — no drug hangover and I'm in control! Using it for 20-40 minutes six nights a week balances my brain the best. Whether I use it for 20 or 40 minutes depends upon how tired I am and whether it's winter or summer.

Nerve Stimulation Units

Zap that pain away! Whether interferential or transcutaneous (TENS), electrical nerve stimulation units can manage pain which may be your constant companion, but is definitely not a friend.

Palm-sized and battery-driven, these devices deliver electrical stimulation to four electrodes that are attached to your body at fleshy, non-hairy locations. The sensation created by the unit works to prevent pain signals from reaching the brain. Though pain relief varies, in many cases the stimulation will greatly reduce or eliminate the pain sensation.

How are the electrode sites selected? What settings can I adjust?
Based on accessibility and nearness to pain and nerve sites, a physical therapist determines optimal placement and pulse settings. Electricity is then channeled to pain-relief sites through electrodes placed directly over or immediately surrounding the painful area.

You can change both the type of pulse and degree of stimulation. For example, one setting sends small comfortable impulses into the painful area, causing a mild tingling sensation. Another causes a muscular contraction. Your physical therapist can show you how to control these.

How fast is pain relief? How long does it last?
Using various pulse settings, such as intermittent or brief and intense, you can feel pain reduction within ten to thirty minutes. If pain is not decreased after sixty minutes, different placement sites are selected.

Pain relief from interferential units usually lasts longer (more than 60 minutes) than with TENS units, although this depends upon the settings, duration of treatment, and unit used. With the TENS setting that produces a muscular contraction, pain relief takes longer to achieve; it also lasts longer (more than an hour) (Kosses, 2004).

Personal experience. I now use an interferential stimulator, which replaced my TENS unit, purchased in the 1990s. Pain relief arrives within a few minutes, especially when an ice pack is applied. It works well — on my terms at my home — for many different kinds of muscular injuries. Lately, it's helping to heal a torn hamstring muscle and continues to help rehab my shoulder after three surgeries. I'm surfing again, so I guess it works! These units also travel well — I took mine to Mexico on a dive trip and the border patrol didn't confiscate it!

Self-Advocacy with Health Professionals

We've all probably done it, one way or another: asked the dentist to fix our broken/sprained ankles or whatever. And, when they told us that it wasn't part of their job description, we huffed out of

> Don't ask the dentist to fix your broken ankle.
> — DJ

there, muttering, "See, no one understands. No one will help me! Brain injury isn't in anyone's job description, and I don't want this job, either!"

But we've got the job, and professionals exist who are able and willing to help us perform to the best of our abilities. Maybe not as much as we want or think we need, as often as we want, as soon as we want, or the way we want.

How do I find survivor-friendly health professionals?

They're out there, the good ones, the ones who'll treat you like a normal person. It just may take a while to connect with them. To link to professionals you'll like and respect, the best way is to ask members of your rewiring teams for referrals to colleagues they like and respect!

How do I communicate with health professionals and their staffs?

The "brain-damaged" or "brain-injury-survivor" label does not usually create respect, so while that's vital information to communicate to the right people, it's counterproductive to tell your story —

> If you don't know where you're going, any road will get you there.
> — Anonymous

what happened, length of time in coma, hospital and rehab settings, how many drugs, etc. — to others who may be working in or visiting the office.

For example, if you trip, fall, and break an ankle, the brain injury may be an indirect cause — you lost your balance and tripped — but your whole history is not required to explain the broken bone! Your brain injury also may or may not affect how the bone is repaired and treated.

Perhaps the ankle break is an indicator — a red flag — of another problem that contributed to your fracture, like an inadequate diet, blood loss, or low calcium absorption, etc. Also, any medications for the broken ankle will affect current meds — and vice versa — so communicate only the appropriate information. Get it?

How Do I Advocate for Myself?

Do's

Before the appointment:

- Discuss the reasons for appointment with family, friends, and your professionals.
- Tape-record or write down questions about diagnosis, treatment options, duration, expected/desired results, and possible side effects.
- Tape-record or write down health history including date of your brain injury, major surgeries, illnesses, and information about both prescribed and over-the-counter medications you take.
- Ask for directions to the office, parking, etc. — and for extra time for questions after your appointment.
- Assemble supplies like a notebook, pen/tape recorder, medical/insurance cards, etc.
- Ask someone to accompany you to help you remember and stay calm.

On the appointment day:

- Allow enough time for relaxed readiness and dress appropriately.
- Eat unless directed not to. If you can't eat before the appointment, bring water and food for later.
- Gather materials and review your notes, questions, and directions.

At the appointment:

- Act respectful and courteous toward the doctor and staff, and your companion.
- Ask relevant questions. Ask the foot doctor about feet, the hand doctor about hands, the head doctor about heads, etc.

- Review what you think they said/meant. Ask, "do you mean…"
- Ask what to do if treatment or drugs don't work.
- Schedule follow-up appointments.

After the appointment:
- Discuss the results of the appointment, treatment options, etc. with others.
- Start treatment recommendations and note changes, positive and/or negative.
- If desired response doesn't occur, call the appointed person (doctor or nurse) to discuss the situation.
- Switch doctors if you don't feel heard.

Don'ts
- Don't act or talk like a victim — don't complain about what "they" did or didn't do.
- Don't discuss irrelevant or unimportant issues like lost benefits, fights with Social Security or your neighbor, etc.
- Don't ask the foot doctor to fix your head or the head doctor to fix your foot!
- Don't go it alone! Many are able and willing to help. Just ask!
- Don't use your cell phone or listen to your iPod or other musical device during the appointment, except while waiting. *Did I need to remind you of this?*
- Don't stop treatment without consultation with someone who knows! Call your doctor or nurse, your pharmacy's 24-hour number, or if necessary, call 911.

Personal experience. Of course I've broken some of the "don't" rules! I also learned that proper preparation and approach saves needless stress. If we prepare medical professionals for their encounters with us, everyone is a winner!

Some thoughts about doctors and our relationships with them.
Doctors choose the medical profession because they feel called to it, especially those who work with survivors. They, too, are often frustrated

with the "system." So, it is even more important to prepare for your visit and show respect. Remember the Golden Rule!

Summary

- Keep looking until you find people you like.
- Be open to different methods, therapies, and devices.
- Trust your gut when choosing therapies and helpers.
- Be prepared for your appointments.
- Don't act or talk like a victim.
- Practice SAFER (Stop, Assess, Fix, Examine, Retry).

> "How many doors do I have to knock on?"
> — me
> "As many as it takes..."
> — Dr. Johnson (DJ)

8

Mind, Body, Spirit Rewiring: Healing with Complementary Therapy

When you have a disease, do not try to cure it.
Find your center, and you will be healed.
— Taoist proverb

In this chapter we look at other therapies that can help you heal including: acupuncture, herbs, manipulation, massage, magnets, and meditation.

Introduction

"How can I heal myself? I'm brain-damaged. Besides, isn't that what doctors are paid to do?"

Sorry — no excuses! Brain-damaged does not mean brain-dead nor does it mean irreparable. While you won't be like you were, you can be better than you are — you can be healthier and happier. And, doctors aren't magicians — they can only help you heal yourself.

Consider the meaning of health. It isn't either the absence of disease or a permanent state of harmony, when body, mind, and spirit are balanced, although we seek those. It also does not mean you'll never be in disharmony; rather, health is the ability to recover from a disharmony, since you and your environment are always changing — that is life!

To help you recover from your injury and rewire, *"there are many paths up the mountain,"* just as there are for your spiritual journey. This chapter explores the complementary treatments that I've experienced or that others recommended. We will look at:

- Traditional Chinese medicine
- Energy healing
- Massage therapy
- Other holistic medical treatments
- Spinal manipulation
- Self-help therapies

Traditional Chinese Medicine

Practiced in China for nearly five thousand years, Traditional Chinese Medicine (TCM) is the granddaddy of recorded holistic medicine and based on the understanding that everything in the world is related. We are all part of this energy-filled universe. In TCM, mind, body, and spirit express different forms of the same life force, *chi* (pronounced "chee"), which is a balance of the two complementary life forces, *yin* and *yang,* that are at work in everything in the universe (Williams, 1996).

Health is a balance of these life forces; disease results if there is either too much or too little of one or the other. Chinese medicine uses the body's energy system to heal and rebalance itself.

What are the differences between Western and Eastern medicine?
Western doctors seek an invading organism as the cause of disease; Chinese doctors look for an imbalance in the body's life forces (Williams, 1996; Moyers, 1993). Many believe that Western medicine is better at trauma care and TCM is better at prevention and healing.

Treating the whole person is the focus of this system. Practitioners focus on prevention, rather than treatment, of disease, and advocate a back-to-basics approach to health. They encourage us to enjoy fresh air and water, plants, sunshine, and regular

> Waiting until you are sick to see a doctor is like waiting until you are thirsty to dig a well.
> — Chinese proverb

exercise. A vital concept is that *chi* (or vital force, or spirit) lives throughout our system and must flow freely to enable our internal healer to work.

Acupuncture

Acupuncture is effective anytime there is a disharmony that results in mental, spiritual, or physical symptoms because it treats their underlying cause. The needling helps to re-establish harmony as it removes blockages of our life force energy, resulting in lasting corrections (Williams, 1996; Moyers, 1993).

What symptoms of brain injury can be helped with acupuncture?

All of them! Because injury weakened your whole body, acupuncture is of special value to you. Besides relieving headache pain, it can also alleviate other chronic pain (due to any cause) because needling mobilizes the body's healing resources to remove the cause of it. Acupuncture speeds healing of soft tissue injuries, diminishes hemi-paralysis, and corrects impaired immune systems and hormonal imbalances (Mac Dorman, 1996; Kaplan, 1998).

Although best known for relief of pain, acupuncture also works for depression and addictions to drugs, alcohol, nicotine, or sugar that are common among survivors, because the involved neurotransmitters can be balanced (Mac Dorman, 1996).

One technique was specially developed for survivors! With the knowledge that all the scalp points represent underlying areas of the brain, a practitioner stimulates the diseased or damaged area to aid a return of function to that area. Scalp acupuncture is especially effective for reducing chronic muscle spasm (Mac Dorman, 1996).

What does an acupuncture diagnosis involve?

A practitioner of Chinese medicine looks, hears, and smells, questions, and touches you to observe where the disharmony exists in your body's energy field. First, a practitioner looks generally at physical appearance and specifically at the tongue, then listens to the sound of the voice and your breathing. Following a series of questions, some of which may seem irrelevant, the physician touches you, generally palpitating the surface of the skin to feel for temperature, body moisture, and any tender spots along the meridians, and then takes your pulse, an especially important diagnostic aspect of Chinese medicine (Williams, 1996).

Acupuncture points relate to organs and provide an easy method of diagnosis; with an imbalance, the corresponding acupuncture point may become tender or red. Stimulating this point influences the circulation of *chi*, and also the related organ and system (Tsuei, 1996).

What does an acupuncture treatment feel like? Is it safe?
A warm sting, like a mosquito bite, is the usual description for a needling sensation. As thin as a hair, stainless steel needles are inserted to a depth of about ¼ inch, depending upon the amount of flesh at the site. When you feel a tingling sensation, the point is accessed. Then the practitioner gently twists or twirls the needle to stimulate the point. Needles remain in for 10-60 minutes, with 20 minutes serving as the average (Williams, 1996). Disposable needles ensure safety.

Location of needles depends on the condition treated; both distant and local points may be used in the same treatment. Diagnostic priorities determine which sites are needled first, and one session may actually involve two separate treatments, with the major disharmony treated first.

Various treatments include electro-acupuncture, where a weak electrical current stimulates needles, and cupping, in which a glass cup is heated to create a vacuum effect and then placed over acupuncture points (Williams, 1996; Moyers, 1993). Specialized tiny needles embedded in a small patch of adhesive may be used for some conditions, like addictions and other chronic states. Needles are placed on ear points and usually remain in place for a week or so, and you press on them for increased effectiveness.

What are reactions and side effects of treatments?
While there are no serious side effects, a few people may experience lightheadedness, which wears off quickly. Most find that treatments are relaxing and many drift into a deep sleep. When the scalp is stimulated, a burning sensation may be felt at the needling point and a dull or numb feeling in the target area (Lewith, 1998).

Following treatments, the typical reaction is tiredness, although some people feel joyful or energized. Some symptoms may feel worse for a short time before they improve. The changes from needling will usually be gradual, although they may be both immediate and dramatic. It is important to know that the degree to which you first respond to the needles does not indicate the effectiveness of a treatment.

Personal experience. Acupuncture works for me! I've relied on it as one of my treatments of choice ever since 1989, when I first tried it with Claudia MacDorman. She treated not only brain-injury-related complaints, but also injury-associated pain and trauma from eye surgeries and numerous sprains and fractures. When I returned for x-rays and follow-up, Western doctors expressed amazement at my rapid healing. Claudia also optimized the function of my compromised immune system, which allowed me to compete in numerous sporting events.

In addition to electro-acupuncture and take-home press-on needles, my treatments included Chinese herbs and commercial tinctures that I rotated year-round to fortify my system. These modalities allowed me to make rigorous demands on my body and brain — at the same time!

I also learned to see an acupuncturist at the first sign of an illness to stop it in its tracks. If I try to fix it on my own and it worsens, more treatments are needed than if seek help right away.

As someone who formerly was so out of balance that I was at the mercy of any practitioner, I now find mind and body harmony that only occasionally, rather than continuously, needs to be balanced,. Since Claudia, I've successfully used acupuncture after other surgeries and injuries, as well as to keep me healthy with the seasons. I'm in my 60s and still racing in triathlons and enjoying many other sports. Try it!

How does acupressure differ from acupuncture?

While they both share the same philosophy and principles of treatment, the difference lies in the suffixes. While acupressure is the application of finger pressure to specific points on the body, acupuncture is penetration of the points with a needle.

> The physician is only nature's assistant.
> — Galen

Both follow the same meridian theory, but needling allows for deeper penetration, and thereby greater benefits. For example, while acupuncture can be used as an anesthetic to block the sharp pain of surgery, acupressure works to alleviate the severe pain of headache. If needling causes you stress, thus reducing the effectiveness of the treatment, acupressure is a good alternative (Williams, 1996).

What is involved with acupressure and what can it treat?
Specific forms of pressure and manipulation are used. Designed to achieve balance between *yin* and *yang* energy, the forms vary from energizing to calming. Pressure is applied with thumb, fingers, or the whole hand to specific points and held for about two to three minutes on each site (Williams, 1996). Acupressure may precede an acupuncture treatment or be used on its own; it is especially helpful for minor disharmonies that involve stagnation of blood or *chi.*

Energy Healing

Like others before them for thousands of years, energy healers use their hands to move and redirect energy flow that is blocked and creating disharmony. Benefits to you include reducing acute or chronic physical and emotional pain and improving other ill-health conditions.

The numerous energy-healing techniques are typically grouped into three basic healing categories: aura, hands-on healing, and massage. Energy healing may be used alone; more typically it is an addition to other treatment modalities, such as chiropractic.

Healing of the Aura

"This sounds far out! What is the aura and do I have one?"

We all radiate a charge. An *aura* is an energy field that exists about five to six inches beyond our physical body. Imagine a full-body halo, like that seen on many pictures of saints (Foley, 2004). Consider people you know who exude anger or glow with joy. Whatever they give out is their aura. What is your aura?

Using her hands, an experienced healer can scan or feel your aura, locate those places where it is torn or damaged, and repair or restore those areas. Invisible to most of us mere mortals, some healers can actually see auras. As they read the body electric, they readjust the charge (Caldecott, 1996; Foley, 2004). Cool, huh? Like hot rewiring!

We'll briefly discuss some ways of redirecting a person's energy.

Qigong

Strong energy from the therapist is transferred — usually without physical contact — through hands moving over a client's body.

Reiki

Energy flows from the practitioners' hands to a client through a series of hand positions on or above the head and shoulders, stomach and feet. Each position is held for three to ten minutes, depending on a client's needs, with treatments lasting between 45 and 90 minutes. *Reiki* (pronounced "ray-kee") treatments are God-driven; practitioners do not direct the healing. *Reiki* heals by charging the affected parts of a client's energy field with positive energy and clearing the negative, which allows the life force to flow in a healthy way (International Center for Reiki Training, 2004). Anxiety and blood pressure can be reduced (Mahoney, 2004).

Hands-on Healing

This section will describe those methods I've experienced:

Jin Shin Jyutsu.

Although the name sounds active like a martial art, you don't have to do anything other than receive. Sounds good, huh?

An ancient art of harmonizing a body's life energy, Jin Shin Jyutsu uses twenty-six "safety energy locks," located along energy pathways, to bring harmony to a body. Following a prescribed order, a practitioner places fingertips on the designated "safety energy locks" in combination to restore energy flow and bring balance to body, mind, and spirit.

Clients remain fully clothed and lie on a padded table in a quiet room (JSJ, 2005). See the Self-Help Healing Treatments section in Chapter 8 for more information.

Personal experience. I first encountered Jin Shin when my network chiropractor, Todd Binkley, asked his wife, Monika, to hold an injured area. It felt better, so she suggested come for a session to learn how to help myself. I practice the "main central" technique, morning and night, to bring harmony. It works!

Three-Heart Balancing.
The originator of this approach is Jaentra Green Gardner. After she was diagnosed with multiple sclerosis, she searched for 22 years to find any method that might help her overcome that illness. Seeking also to help others heal themselves, Gardner incorporated her many years of learning into this method, which focuses on the teamwork of healer, recipient, and God. Although "three-heart" could refer to the preceding three partners, to Gardner, it refers to the balance in the gravitational field in our bodies of what is called our "third eye" in the middle of the forehead, our physical heart, and our seat of *chi*, just below the navel. Three-Heart Balancing principles include: "Healing is teamwork. We healed you; not I healed you.", "Every act of healing is an act of praying.", and "When love goes in, emotions flow freely." (Gardner, 2000).

What happens in a session?
Fully clothed, you lie on a padded table for one to three hours, as a practitioner gently lays her hands on you. Healers often work in a team of two or more, with one at your head and one at your feet. While practitioners and recipients both typically feel heat and intensity, only the healers' hands feel pain or other uncomfortable sensations. These are released by removing the hands from the client's body and simply shaking them, carefully avoiding the client! Bad energy be gone!

How can energy healing help survivors?
Do you want to lose the pain in your head and other body parts? Healers in my friend Marlys' group found that not only did stroke survivors dramatically improve mobility and function in their activities of daily living (ADLs), but also that the formerly restrictive pain substantially subsided or disappeared! How's that for help?

Personal experience. When my best friend, Marlys Henke, first became interested and began practicing energy healing, even I was somewhat skeptical. But I became a believer when she visited and worked on me nearly every day for about a week. Suddenly, I began to multitask, something I'd been unable to do since my injury 24 years earlier! And feeling the energy flow is nothing less than amazing.

That summer when I visited her, Marlys invited me to partner with her as we worked on others; helping people is an awesome feeling. Recently, I experienced the power of this method again. Still feeling constant pain from major shoulder surgery, I traveled to Minnesota for a high school reunion and stayed with Marlys for over three weeks. She worked on me every night and during the day if I felt pain. After only five days, I stopped all pain medication because the unremitting ache and pain were gone! The third day was the most powerful when four healers worked on me for over an hour. I'm still pain-free!

Massage Therapy

"Ahhh — this feels so good!" is a typical response for anyone who's experienced the soothing pleasures of massage. We know it's a potent stress reliever, but why does it feel so good? Massage stimulates the brain to produce endorphins, which control pain. It is a healing art on all three levels: physical, mental, and spiritual.

What are the different kinds of massage?
Most people associate massage with "Swedish massage," in which a therapist uses oil to assist the flow of long, gliding strokes. Some kneading and friction on the upper layers of muscles may also be included, but the goal usually is relaxation, not stimulation. Acupressure was discussed earlier. Here we talk about shiatsu and reflexology.

Shiatsu
This is the Japanese form of pressure-point massage in which a practitioner concentrates on the specific acupuncture points that feel like nodules under the skin when pressed. To us, the nodule feels like a trigger point — it may be hot and sensitive. However, pressure on the site is usually experienced as therapeutic pain — the kind that is needed to heal (Williams, 1996). Using only hands and fingers to apply pressure to these specified points, Shiatsu practitioners stimulate circulation in the body's systems.

By deeply massaging the muscles, fatigue-producing metabolic waste products are eliminated and general good health is promoted. To prevent and cure illness is the goal of shiatsu, which may also use movement and stretching (Namikoshi, 1981).

Reflexology
Stimulating over 7000 nerve endings in each foot, practitioners of reflexology use only their thumbs and fingers to massage the feet. Designed to improve circulation, and thereby increase energy and help achieve homeostasis, working on the hands and feet has been practiced throughout the ages by the Orientals and Egyptians.

The healing art of reflexology, as it is known today, is based on the theory that specific points in the feet and hands correspond to all the glands and organs in the body. These points respond to the stimulus of touch, thus the term *reflex* (Horton, 1998).

Personal experience. While work on feet can be painful, it is also a relief. As an athlete, my feet are always under pressure to perform, and they frequently voice their need for attention. Massaging them so relaxes and rejuvenates me that I feel the "ahh" throughout my entire body! Although I've not sought a reflexology-only treatment, my massage therapist always kneads my feet and hands, and I use a wooden roller every night to stimulate reflexology points. It feels so good when I stop!

How does massage work?
Physically, massage increases blood and lymphatic flow throughout the body, reduces edema (swelling), loosens scar tissue, removes waste products, and delivers nutrients. Massage also gently stretches muscles, which helps to normalize our metabolic processes and increase joint range of motion so we don't become stiff and unable to move. It tones the reflexive actions of nerves so they can respond to a stimulus like a hot flame; and it lubricates and stimulates the sensory receptors of our skin, enhancing cell turnover and sloughing off dead cells.

Mentally, the healing touch of massage not only improves our brain function by increasing blood flow, but also helps us to think more clearly by relaxing nerves and muscles and reducing stress hormones — this makes us smarter!

Spiritual and emotional well-being are also enhanced by the physical touch. Therapists can transfer their positive healing energy to us and their hands communicate care and compassion, comforting jangled nerves.

How can massage improve health?
If you've ever had one, you don't need to ask, but there are several important ways that massage can aid your rewiring journey.

Massage aids healing of the massive physical injuries that usually accompany a brain injury. In addition to reducing stress hormones, massage can help restore joint mobility by relaxing soft tissue, improve blood flow to introduce nutrients and remove waste products that allows tissue to heal. If limbs are inactive, blood flow is impaired. Massage mechanically assists muscles in their effort to regain the chemical balance that is disturbed with inactivity (Tappan, 1998).

Many of us sustain lower back injuries as well as neck and head injuries. Combining massage with pressure on trigger points can significantly reduce both chronic and acute lower back pain as well as increasing muscle flexibility and tone. The tension headaches that seem to plague all of us can be relieved by massage of head, neck, and shoulder areas. Other benefits include relieving withdrawal symptoms of alcohol addiction and speeding wound healing. Used as a treatment for insomnia, massage is also effective at reducing anxiety and coping with hospital stress (Moline, 1998). All this — plus it feels so good!

Other Holistic Medical Treatments

Homeopathy and how survivors might benefit.
Treating the whole person as well as a specific condition, homeopathy aims to raise general health to reduce susceptibility to disease, without the harmful side effects of conventional drugs. Practitioners believe that our body develops symptoms as a way to heal itself.

A homeopathic physician can correct profound imbalances and build a strong immune system in us by treating our individual pattern of reactions from a holistic view (Dannheisser & Edwards, 1998).

Those who are affected with balance disorders could benefit from a homeopathic medication, Vertigoheel, which is effective for vertigo symptoms. It is considered to be as safe as a standard drug, betahistine — this was the first time the American Medical Association (AMA) published study results of a homeopathic remedy (Heel, 1998)

Personal experience. In response to a sudden onset of flu symptoms (sneezing, chills, fever, muscle aches) and the unavailability of my acupuncturist, I tried a homeopathic remedy, Oscillococcinum.

With a three-dose regimen, it would work either fast or not at all. As the first dose dissolved under my tongue, I rested, prepared a salad, went to the movies, ate dinner, took another dose, and went to bed. During the night when I awakened, I took another dose. The next morning I worked at the computer and took a short bike ride. Later, feeling better, I went for an easy three-mile run at low tide. Although I took it easy, the remedy worked, because I stayed symptom-free. This demands a repeat!

Osteopathy and what it offers survivors

While doctors evaluate the whole person, this system focuses on the musculoskeletal system, which reflects and influences all other interconnected body systems. Observing how our bodies function, hands-on manipulation may be used as physicians seek to improve circulation and restore normal balance to our body and structure. Doctors also discuss lifestyle factors and emphasize diet and exercise as preventative measures of health care (Bezilla, 1997).

With the shock to our system and our bodies out of balance, we are good candidates for the technique of craniosacral therapy. This manual method, specific to cranial osteopathy, is designed to remove the functional restrictions and associated symptoms that are caused by soft tissue injuries, especially cranial and sacral (Feeley, 1998).

Spinal manipulation/chiropractic

Spinal manipulation, often called an adjustment, has been used for thousands of years in many different cultures; evidence of manipulative therapy, exercise, and massage is seen in ancient drawings. Some hieroglyphics depict back walking and the use of crude devices to stretch and correct spinal abnormalities.

Chiropractic has refined these techniques. The word *chiro* means "hand"; *practic* means "treatment" or "practice"; *chiropractic* means "hand treatment." The goal is to correct nerve interference and the malfunctioning that result from improper alignment of the spine. Chiropractors unlock and release vertebrae from their misaligned positions (Rondberg, 1996). The most common treatment is for back problems, but chiropractors also work on other parts of the spine and joints.

How can chiropractic help survivors of traumatic brain injuries?

Does you neck hurt? How about your head? Probably both if you're a survivor. The cause may be from whiplash injury. Chiropractic care can decrease your pain and significantly increase flexibility and strength. One study found that 80% of headaches are due to misalignment of the cervical spine (ACA, 1998).

Chiropractors are skilled at providing long-term headache relief and it lasts longer than an aspirin (or ten) or other medications, such as antidepressants, with no dry mouth, drowsiness, or weight gain!

Other chiropractic/manipulative techniques

In addition to spinal manipulation, other specialized kinds of treatment performed by chiropractors, osteopaths, naturopaths, massage therapists, and others can be a boon to survivors. See Chapter 8 in *Brain Injury Rewiring for Loved Ones* to learn about them.

Personal experience. After thirty years, I'm still getting better and my muscles still respond to changes. Some years ago, I began to see a different chiropractor, who was appalled at the difference in my leg lengths. His practice included a different kind of cervical neck work that releases the structure to allow a short leg to lengthen. I tried it; it worked. My short leg, which formerly was nearly ½ inch shorter, is now almost the same length. No more orthotics (shoe inserts) for me as well as no pain, plus better form and improved times. Best of all, running is no longer the ordeal it was after my injury — now I love to run!

Self-Help Healing Treatments

Many of us are do-it-yourselfers; we like to learn a technique so we can use it whenever we need it. To help heal yourself, depending on your style, there are several options: ask questions of your health professionals, observe therapists in action, attend a seminar taught by a practicing clinician, and/or find resources at the library or bookstore.

We'll start with imagery, move on to the traditional Chinese medicine (TCM) system of self-healing, then we'll discuss Jin Shin Jyutsu, imaging, and meditation techniques, followed by magnetic therapy.

How can these techniques benefit survivors? Besides being simple to do, how about more energy, less stress, and better health?

Imagery Techniques

Remember how different musical sounds can energize, relax, depress, and cheer us? What we picture in our minds can do the same things. Pay attention to your body as you imagine yourself standing on the median on a crowded freeway. Then, to escape that frenzied state, place yourself on a beach or in a canoe on a calm lake — or wherever you choose!

In the first scene, your nervous system prepared you to fight or flee the freeway, then your body and mind tensed for action. In the second scene, you felt the peace of the water and relaxed. What we imagine influences our body's responses.

If we picture pain as a fire, a knife, or an animal, we can use our imagination to explore like a camera might, and see how to remove the source of the pain and also what caused it. We can picture a firefighter extinguishing flames, a police officer handcuffing a crazed knife-wielder, or a trainer subduing an animal. We can see good soldiers gobbling up bad germs. Our medicines find their targets and our treatments zap the enemy. When the pain returns, our forces return to conquer it.

Another way to use guided imagery is the inner advisor technique. Picture a wise person who is ready to help solve the problem — maybe a higher power or an angel or just someone insightful. After you share your dilemma, not only will you feel a sense of peace, but also hear an obvious solution. Allowing our creative selves a voice lightens emotional burden and provides new insights.

Healing can begin when we analyze our imaginings and choose how we'll use what we saw. To successfully do this, many of us need help. To learn about therapist-directed guided imagery and hypnosis, see Chapter 8 in *Brain Injury Rewiring for Loved Ones*.

Self-Healing from Chinese Medicine

How's your *chi*? As you may recall, Chinese medicine uses the body's energy system to heal itself, to rebalance and to restore your energy flow. To learn how to move it yourself, here are four techniques that can be done in any position of your choice: lying, sitting, or standing:

Deep Breathing

Take a slow deep breath through your nose, filling your lungs completely. Exhale slowly for 10 seconds, either silently or audibly, relaxing deeply each time. Repeat frequently during the day, developing a pattern of deep breathing. Perhaps use the signal of a telephone or a red light or before eating to remind yourself to breathe deeply. Maybe even smile as you do it!

Gentle Movement

Stand with feet shoulder width apart, arms relaxed. Bend your knees slightly, moving your tailbone beneath your spine to lengthen your back and slow your energy. Slowly inhale as you face your palms forward and rise onto the balls of your feet, raising your arms with palms up to shoulder height, keeping elbows slightly bent. Slowly exhale as you face your palms downward and slowly lower your arms, returning your heels to the floor. Swing your hands back slightly as they pass your legs, gently lifting your toes. As you develop a gentle rhythm, repeat 10-15 times or as tolerated, building up to 15 times.

Self-Massage

Start with the hands: from any position, apply gentle pressure with your left thumb to the palm of your right hand, supporting your remaining fingers on the back of the right hand. Gradually increase the pressure. Massage your whole hand, including fingers, noting tender areas. Holding each finger, pinch gently on both sides of the nail simultaneously. Switch hands and repeat the process. Return to any tender spots and gently knead. Move to the internal organs to warm and energize them: Place your palms on the lower edge of your rib cage, near the sides of your body. Rub your palms in a circular motion against your body, breathing easily and deeply. Do you feel the warmth your hands generate? Next place one hand on your breastbone and the other on your navel. Rub in a circular motion with each hand. Now move your hands to your lower back and repeat the process. Do as often as you please!

Mindfulness

In a technique called mindfulness, we focus on a single bodily sensation, which prevents worry from entering our minds and frees us from stress. As you breathe through your nostrils, focus all your attention on the feeling of the air as it passes through them, cool on the inhale and warm as it exhales. Repeat once or as long as you like up to about 20 minutes. If you do it any longer, you'll probably fall asleep!

Using these four techniques for just 10-15 minutes daily promises to improve energy, reduce vulnerability to illness and the negative effects of stress. One idea is to do them all as you awaken each morning and before you sleep each evening (Jahnke, 1997). *It works for me!*

Self-Help Acupressure

Did you ever apply pressure with your thumb to a sore muscle? Did you find relief? That's acupressure! Pushing on a painful area may be a natural response — pain invites us to act. Pressure-point therapy is especially effective with headaches and nausea.

Traditional Chinese medicine says that when we apply pressure to an area, we strengthen *chi*, and when we add a small rotating motion to the pressure, we move and reduce blocked bioenergy. Western medicine believes the benefits of acupressure come from stimulating the brain to release endorphins (Gach, 1997).

How can self-help acupressure benefit brain injury survivors?

How about reduced muscular tension, increased circulation, and relief of pain? Ever need headache relief or an unclouded mind? Just apply pressure for two to three minutes on hand, neck, or head points.

Let's start with the easiest place, the hand. The headache point is in the web of skin between the thumb and forefinger. Firm thumb pressure is applied to one hand, then to the other. You feel better fast!

Let's move on to the head points. One head point is between the eyebrows in the middle of the forehead, where gentle finger pressure is applied. Pressure on this point can clear the mind as well as reduce headache! For an alternative, apply simultaneous pressure on two points: with one hand, press the hollow in the back of your neck at the base of the skull at the same time as you press into the upper hollows of the eye sockets with thumb and forefinger with the other hand. Use the same firm but gentle pressure on the other head points, over the temple area. Neck points can be found on both sides of the spinal column.

For other sore areas, use firm and stationary pressure from your thumb or middle finger for two to three minutes per site. If acupuncture points are located on both sides of the body, apply pressure to one side, then to the other. If the points are sensitive to the touch, you've located the correct spots! (Gach, 1997)

Personal experience. As an athlete, I've known about acupressure points for years — but just didn't call them that. When I had a sore muscle, I'd instinctively push on the area. It felt better, so I kept doing it. When I had ulcers, pushing on the pain relieved it. I acquired the acupressure charts to learn how to do it myself. Now, when I feel soreness or pain, I can apply what I know first, and then go to one of my healers if I can't fix it. With basic knowledge, when I seek help from a professional, I can ask technical questions, observe what they do, and maybe the next time, do it myself!

Jin Shin Jyutsu

Want to harmonize your energy every day? Then follow this series of nine hand positions:

Hold each position until energy (pulsation) is felt.

1. Place your right hand on top of your head, maintaining this position throughout the routine.
2. Place your left fingers (or finger) between your eyebrows.
3. Move your left fingers to the tip of your nose.
4. Place your left fingers on the "V" of your neck.
5. Place your left fingers on the center of your breastplate (sternum).
6. Move your left fingers to base of breastplate.
7. Measuring approximately one inch above the navel, place your left fingers on this area.
8. Move your left fingers to your pubic bone and simultaneously
9. Move your right hand to the base of your spine.

At the beginning, this routine may take a minute or two, but as the sensation becomes more and more familiar, feeling the energy is almost instantaneous. If any step is uncomfortable to reach, go to the next step (JSJ, 2005).

How can Jin Shin help survivors?

Not only does it harmonize energy, it also balances emotions. Who doesn't need that? And, this technique is so discrete it may be done anywhere, anytime; your friends and family will love it, too. For worry, wrap your right hand around your left thumb. Hold and repeat with other hand. If fearful, surround your index finger with your hand. OK, now for my favorite: Guess which finger is the anger finger? Yep, it's the third finger! Wrap it with your right hand. Some people may find it necessary to alternate hands to obtain the maximum effect with this one! For sadness/grief, wrap the fourth (ring) finger and for anxiety, the fifth (baby) finger (JSJ, 2005).

Personal experience. Ever since Monika Binkley taught me this procedure, I do it morning and night while still in bed. It is a good way for me to begin and end the day!

Hands-On Healing

Want another way to remove pain by yourself? Place one or both hands on the pain area or place one hand on your heart. Experiment and see what works best. It works even better if a loved one can lend a hand, because the energy of two is stronger. Also, when someone else is touching us, they can remove the energy and discard it!

Magnetic Therapy

Block pain by a magnet held against the skin of a painful area? Yep, and we're not talking voodoo or virtual medicine here, but another new discovery of an old remedy.

How do magnets work? Several theories explain the magic of this energy medicine: increasing blood flow speeds healing and prevents muscle spasms; the slight electrical current created by the magnetic field stimulates the nervous system and either triggers the blockage of pain sensations or the release of endorphins, your body's natural pain relievers (Poirot, 1998); and magnet therapy assists the body to regain its self-healing balance naturally (Wiancko, 1995).

How can magnets help survivors? What kinds of magnets work?

Got pain? Studies find that approximately 80% of people who suffer from chronic pain of any kind can be helped with magnetic therapy — with no side effects (Lawrence, 1998). Any painful area where a magnet could be taped to the skin is a target. Ears have a large number of acupuncture points and are good sites. If a magnet placed directly over the pain site isn't effective after a few days, then use several magnets located at acupuncture points that correspond to that pain. Even those who suffer from depression may be offered magnetic therapy in the near future, as success has been reported in small studies (La Voie, 1997).

As with every type of treatment, individual responses to magnets vary. Some people are sensitive and can feel the magnets in a few minutes; others may take days. Experiment!

We're not talking refrigerator magnets here; their strength is only about 10 gauss, too weak to penetrate the skin and provide any benefits. Medical magnets range from about 450 gauss to 10,000 gauss, with the higher number offering more pain relief (Altman 1997).

The more user-friendly, the more it costs. Magnets may be attached with adhesive tape, encased in a pad or wrap, or worn as a piece of jewelry. Wraps, bands, bracelets, necklaces, cushions and mattresses contain a number of powerful magnets, thus maximizing their strength.

Meditation

We've all seen pictures of people sitting cross-legged, eyes closed, with their palms raised and hands resting on their legs — symbols of tranquility. While sitting quietly in the yoga lotus position is a traditional pose, many different meditation methods can benefit us.

Meditating includes repeating a sound, phrase, or motion, while ignoring all other sounds, thoughts, or activities. Beads or other aids may be used. The keys to meditation are natural breathing and concentration — whether on your breathing, a mantra, a motion, or a physical point. A mantra is a sound that generally has no verbal meaning. Its purpose is to still the mind, operate as a healing power, and keep distracting thoughts away. Some examples include: "peace," "Love," "Om," "thank you."

How do I meditate?

You can sit, stand, recline, chant, garden, run, paddle, swim, cycle, roll, walk, pray, dance, wash dishes, maybe just breathe deeply — repeat any sound or activity and focus on it. There is no one correct way to meditate; experiment with what works best for you. This may vary because we are all in a state of flux! Books and classes may help; CDs are especially useful. Trust your instincts and select what works. Practice at home — at your own pace. Digestion interferes with the process, so meditate either before meals or two hours after meals.

For a sitting meditation, choose a quiet environment in a warm location. Sit quietly in a comfortable position, wearing non-binding clothing. Close your eyes. If your muscles are not relaxed, consciously loosen all of them, starting with your feet and ending with your face. Maintain this relaxed state. Slowly and deeply breathe through your nose, silently repeating the number "one" or another mantra as you breathe out. Meditate for 10 to 20 minutes; even five minutes provides some benefits. After you finish, continue to sit quietly, breathing deeply, for a few minutes, starting with your eyes closed.

How do I know if I'm doing it right?

If you feel comfortable and find the peace you seek, it's working. Even if your mind isn't still all the time, if you can bring it back to that place of quiet, keep practicing the same way. Just because it's a discipline doesn't mean it's something to endure — it's meant to be gratifying!

If, on the other hand, it just doesn't feel right, perhaps a change would help. Maybe alter how you meditate, your mantra, setting, or time of day. Then try again! Keep changing until it feels right and you get the results you want. Remember SAFER: Stop, Assess, Fix, Examine, Retry.

If intrusive thoughts interfere, acknowledge them and then let them pass, as you return to your mantra. Repeat this technique in the same place at least once a day to develop the habit. With practice, relaxation will come more readily, and the internal chatter will gradually be replaced by silence. Experts say that we must learn to meditate, just as we learned to walk. And, if we expect more difficulty maintaining our meditative state during periods of stress, it won't add to our stress!

How does meditation heal? How can meditation help survivors?
Meditation decreases muscle tension, so our bodies need less energy, which slows breathing and lowers stress-related hormones, protecting us against anxiety and depression. It can even help us control our anger because minor things won't upset us as much (Benson, 1998). Alleviating pain, especially chronic pain that has not responded to standard medical treatment, can be a major benefit for us. Various studies show that those who meditate experience reduced pain, whether from muscle tension, headache, or other conditions. Healing the mind changes the body. Some studies also show improved functioning of the right hemisphere of the brain, which is associated with creativity and imagination (Redwood, 1998).

Summary

Now that you know many paths up the healing mountain, I hope that you investigate the ones that appeal to you, knowing that something, somewhere will resonate with you. May God bless your journey!

> Any path is only a path, and there is no affront, to oneself or to others, in dropping it if that is what your heart tells you.
> — Carlos Castaneda

9
Nutritional Rewiring: Healing with Healthy Eating and Lifestyle

You are what you eat.

— Adelle Davis

In this chapter we will look at the importance nutrition and lifestyle on our rewiring. We need healthy food to support our bodies in the healing process. As we live each day, good food is one of the keys to optimizing our ability to be at our best.

Introduction

"Right, lady. Let's see if I get this. In the Spiritual Rewiring chapter you tell me I can heal my brain injury with prayer and the arts, like God and Mozart. Okay, I can do that. I believe in God and I like music. But now you tell me I can heal my body with the food I eat? Yes! This I gotta hear! I knew colas and burgers were good for me."

Well, yes, burgers can fit into a healthy diet and a cola now and then is okay — if you eat lots of fruits and veggies and downsize the large order of fries. Did you know that our bodies hunger for nutritious food and that we can boost our brainpower just by eating? Let's learn how.

"I'll get hungry if I digest a whole chapter on food!"

Not if you eat first. So, to nurture your neurons, hunker down with a cup of tea or coffee, a chunk of dark chocolate, almonds, and fresh apple slices. Then turn on your tunes and ready your receivers. Here goes!

Nutritional Rewiring examines how your food not only charges your cells now, but also repairs injured connections and guards against future damage. To optimize your immune system functioning, you will learn how to make wise choices to ensure that what you eat is not only good to eat — but also good for you! We also review fast-food charts to make healthy eating work for us in the real world.

We consider the special dietary needs of survivors and explain simple ways to meet them. We answer questions like "Do comfort foods fit in my diet plan?" and "Can I eat fast food in a healthy diet?" We simplify food labels and examine such misunderstood concepts as free radicals, antioxidants, Daily Value, Required Daily Allowance (RDA), serving size, calories, metabolic rate, good and bad fat, and cholesterol. We talk about chocolate, caffeine, and brain food, and we demonstrate how to use a new government nutrition site (www.MyPyramid.gov). You will also learn about sugar cravings and addictions, how sleep helps our brains recover, and how and why to get our crucial Zs! In this chapter we discuss:

- What is nutrition?
- Why is optimal nutrition important?
- Why do I need vitamins and minerals?
- How do I develop a healthful eating plan?
- Nutrition questions and answers.
- Healthy lifestyle habits.

Nutrition Basics

Nutrition is the study of how our bodies use the food that fuels our daily activities. As such, "my body, my car" is a useful concept to keep in mind when we think about our nutritional needs. Let's consider fuel.

> Every day you do one of two things: build health or produce disease in yourself.
> — Adelle Davis

What kinds of fuel do our bodies use?
Different kinds of fuels provide different amounts of nutrients and calories (energy) for us to use. Some fuels, like soft drinks or colas, give us short-lived energy and no nutrients. These are called empty calories. Foods like fish, eggs, nuts, and seeds, are nutrient-dense; they are powerful building and maintaining sources. Other food is calorie-dense, providing lots of energy for its size. High-fat food like nuts and seeds or high-sugar food like raisins are dense in both calories and nutrients.

What nutrients compose this fuel?
Our food contains six types of nutrients: proteins, carbohydrates, fats, vitamins, minerals, and water — often called the "forgotten nutrient."

Proteins are used to build, maintain, and repair tissue in our brains and bodies, including neurotransmitters. Some protein is also converted into energy. Composed of building blocks of amino acids, every living cell in our body contains protein in the outer and inner membranes. Muscle, bone, and red blood cells, in particular, contain a lot of protein.

Carbohydrates give us energy, fiber, and nutrients. Composed of various types of sugar that provide the primary fuel for our bodies, carbohydrates also regulate the amount of circulating sugar in our blood, and assist in calcium absorption.

Fats provide energy, help our bodies absorb vitamins, keep our skin glowing, and our hair glossy. Fats also give us a feeling of fullness after eating by slowing digestion. Some dietary fats are used to make tissue and manufacture biochemicals like hormones and neurotransmitters. Others transport hormones and fat-soluble vitamins. Not only is our brain about half fat, but essential body fat protects and insulates our internal organs, cushions our skin, and gives shape to our bodies.

How do I know if a food is a carbohydrate, protein, or fat?
Think about what it does for you. If it provides quick energy, it's mostly carbohydrate (fruits, vegetables, grains). If it mostly builds or repairs and usually walks or swims, it's protein (fish, meat, dairy). Tofu, eggs, dry beans and peas, nuts and seeds, are also proteins, but watch out if they grow legs! If it tastes rich and provides a feeling of fullness, it's likely high in fat (nuts, butter, ice cream, some cheese, pastries). Fat also

supplies slow-burning energy and works with protein and carbohydrates to fuel us for our endurance (longer than one hour) activities.

How much fuel do carbohydrates, fats, and protein contain?

All food contains calories that give us energy that our bodies can either use for current work or store for later use. All three kinds of food sources provide energy. Carbohydrates (carbs) provide our main energy source because they are most readily burned. Proteins are burned next. Fats take the longest time to break down in our bodies, so provide a long-lasting fuel source. Fat also needs carbs to burn (fat burns in a carbohydrate flame).

Some foods are denser (contain more calories) than others. To measure how much energy (in calories) is available, we weigh the food in a unit called a gram. Fats contain nine calories per gram (40 calories per teaspoon), alcohol gives us seven calories per gram, and carbohydrates and proteins provide four calories per gram.

It's easy to consume a lot of calories when food and drinks are high in fat and sugar. Some examples: premium ice cream is high in both fat and sugar, movie-theater popcorn and many salad dressings are high in fat, and coffee drinks may contain hidden fats and sugars that can make them very high-calorie.

How can I know the amount of fuel in my food?

Protein sources (meat, fish, dairy, nuts, and dried beans) are important because your body needs proteins to rewire. To select the right protein sources it is important to look at the amount of fat that comes along with the protein.

For meat, the best way to find low-fat meats is to look at the meat itself. If you can't see any fat, as with lean round steak, then the fat content actually is low. A four-ounce serving of lean round steak has about 26 grams of protein and only four grams of fat. Twenty-percent-fat hamburger is another story. It has about 24 grams of protein, but it comes with 18 grams of fat. For chicken and turkey, the dark meat has more fat than the light meat, and the skin is the part with even more fat.

Fish can be high or low in fat, but the omega-3 oil in fatty fish is the good kind that we need. Nuts are also high in fat, but, as with fish, the fat is healthy. Dairy products vary based on the amount of milk fat added. Skim milk is fat free and sour cream is almost all fat. Some people think of tofu as a low-fat food, but the real numbers for a four-ounce serving are nine grams of protein and almost five grams of fat.

Vegetables and fruits provide only a tiny amount of fat and variable amounts of carbohydrates. For example, lettuce and broccoli are low in carbohydrates but white potatoes and bananas are high.

Grains offer only a small amount of fat and significant sugars, but the carbohydrate in whole grains is complex, which is the good kind because it digests slowly to help us maintain a steady source of energy. Examples include: oatmeal, brown rice, and whole grain bread. Avoid grains with added sugar and bread that lists refined flour first. Nutrition labels are very useful for seeing what is really in our food. The ingredient labels help, too, since the ingredients are listed with the largest amounts first.

What are the best kinds of fat to consume? What kinds to avoid?
Most foods contain some fat, so choose good fat over bad fat foods.

Good fats: In addition to the polyunsaturated omega-3 fat found in fish, the best kind of fat to consume is the kind found in avocados, nuts, and unsaturated vegetable oils. These oils include monounsaturated canola, olive, and peanut oils, and polyunsaturated soy, corn, and sunflower oils.

Bad fats are hazardous to your health. They raise cholesterol levels (especially LDL), clog arteries, and lead to strokes and heart attacks. The two basic kinds are (1) saturated fat, found in animal products (butter, lard, red meat) and tropical oils (like coconut and palm that are used in flavoring) and (2) trans fat, found in fast foods, processed foods, packaged baked goods, mayonnaise, stick margarine, and hydrogenated or partially hydrogenated vegetable shortening.

Trans-fatty acids are sneaky, in that they start as liquid and then are hardened through a chemical process (hydrogenation) into a solid. They not only raise the bad LDL cholesterol blood levels, but they lower the good HDL levels! Our bodies find it hard to break down these fats, so they hang around to cause trouble, like increasing heart disease risk. Trans fat is being eliminated but check food labels to be sure!

How can I remember which foods are high in fat and/or sugar?
Foods that are high in fat and sugar are often the ones we find the tastiest. Fat makes food taste good, so choose just a few fatty foods as treats in your daily diet. If it tastes sweet, it's sweetened with either sugar or artificial sweeteners. Foods that are high in both fat and sugar include baked goods, ice cream, and coffee drinks. Some foods high in bad fat (saturated and trans-fat) and bad (simple sugar) carbs include:

- Most fast food.
- Commercially fried and deep-fried foods like doughnuts.
- Most red meat, especially sausage.
- Processed/packaged foods.
- Lard, which may be used in fast food.
- Regular chips, crackers, pretzels.
- Movie-theater and some microwave popcorn.
- Many cereals. Check package for sugar content.
- Some dairy products like cream, ice cream, butter, cheese, some yogurts.
- Packaged baked goods like cookies, cakes, pies, muffins, bagels.
- Sugar-sweetened sodas and fruit drinks.
- Candy and other sweets.
- Some energy bars.

Personal experience. I used to love to eat potato chips — until I discovered their fat content! I tried rice cakes, but the Styrofoam flavor didn't appeal to me, so I went chip-less until the development of tasty low-fat potato and corn chips. Now, I savor each bite!

Optimal Nutrition

Our bodies and brains need a healthy diet to recover from our injuries. We need to rebuild damaged cells, replenish nutrients that are rapidly used for repair, and guard against accelerated "rusting."

Do you remember that brain injury may be called "instant aging?" Not only did our injuries move us into the fast lane as far as the normal oxidative processes that occur as we age, but we lost brain tissue, too.

Injured brains are also more at risk from *free radicals*. These cell-damaging chemicals — formed at injury and from daily living activities like eating and breathing — create havoc, especially with weakened cells.

What we eat significantly impacts aging conditions, neutralizes *free radicals,* and is the most important contributor to the health of our immune systems. Do you want your medications to work? Do you want to feel good? Then eat healthy food! Remember: junk in, junk out.

What kinds of foods boost my brainpower and heal my body?

You've probably heard about the brain-bolstering powers of fish. If you wonder why they're so special, it's because our lipid ratios (balance of fats) are more similar to that of tropical fish and shellfish than any other known food source (Broadhurst et al., 1998). As we evolved — and ate more fish — research suggests that our fatty brains grew smarter!

So to help repair your brain, guard against damage, and boost its power, eat fish at least twice a week, especially fresh, cold-water, oily fish (e.g., salmon, halibut, sea bass, rainbow trout, swordfish, oysters, mackerel), canned herring, sardines, and tuna.

Other ways to obtain this omega-3 kind of fat every include eating nuts (like walnuts, almonds, pistachios, sesame seeds, pecans, ground flaxseed), and taking a supplement. To avoid spoilage, refrigerate these.

Another way to safeguard thinking skills, especially your memory, is to eat at least three cups of vegetables every day, especially green leafy varieties, like spinach. Why? Vegetables contain high amounts of Vitamin E and leafy greens are typically eaten with added fats, such as salad dressing and seeds, which increase vitamin E absorption. Eat a variety of greens and experiment with different ones in combination.

What's the story on *antioxidants* and *free radicals*?

Daily living creates *free radicals*. When you breathe, oxygen reacts with other body compounds to release energy. This oxidation continuously creates *free radicals*. Atoms moving between molecules is one of the processes that provides energy for out bodies. When atoms recombine, they will sometimes get into situations where the molecule is missing an electron. A molecule with a missing electron is a *free radical*.

Normally the situation is handled by antioxidants, which are also part of normal body processes. *Antioxidants* can supply an extra electron without becoming *free radicals* themselves. Problems occur when there are not enough *antioxidants*. Then the free radicals grab electrons from other molecules. If that happens to be part of the cell wall of the DNA, cells can be damaged enough to become cancerous or die. Cells do have mechanisms to repair some damage, but *free radical* damage can add up.

The *free radicals* break down cells, weaken the immune system, deteriorate joints, and promote heart disease and cancer. They also speed oxidation of bad cholesterol (low-density lipoprotein or LDL), which causes accumulation of cholesterol along artery walls and can lead to heart attack or stroke. *Free radicals* damage insulin-producing beta cells in the pancreas, promoting diabetes. More brain cells are also damaged, which leads to degenerative neurological disease processes like Parkinson's and Alzheimer's. Whew! What a hit list!

How do antioxidants fight free radicals?

To neutralize *free radicals* and protect our cells we need antioxidants. Our bodies naturally produce some *antioxidants* compounds and we get others from our foods. The most important of the compounds in food are vitamin E, beta-carotene, and vitamin C. The *antioxidants* stop free radicals, repair cellular damage, act as anti-inflammatories, and boost the immune system.

Colorful produce is a rich source of these compounds. With the exception of mushrooms, cauliflower, and onions, color is a good clue to a food's nutritional value — the deeper the shade, the healthier.

To choose, picture the variety and vivid colors in an artist's paint box: red, green, blue, orange, and yellow. Consider the differences among leafy green varieties, like iceberg lettuce, spinach, and romaine. Iceberg is pale green and provides little nutritional value. Spinach, on the other hand, is rich dark green and full of antioxidants. Romaine lettuce is also a good choice, both for its antioxidant properties and for high fiber content.

Vitamins and Minerals

Vitamins help regulate work within cells and affect all functions in our bodies. Although only tiny amounts of these substances are needed to perform their tasks, they are absolutely essential to human life. They do not supply energy, but some of them (the B vitamins) help convert food to energy. Others serve as scavengers and destroy rampaging free radicals. These internal guardian nutrients include Vitamins C and E, carotenoids, and the minerals iron, zinc, and selenium.

Vitamins are categorized as either fat-soluble (Vitamins A, D, E, or K) or water-soluble (B vitamins or Vitamin C). Our bodies store fat-soluble vitamins for relatively long periods, but water-soluble vitamins remain in the body for only a short time, so need to be replenished frequently. Otherwise, deficiencies develop within weeks, such as scurvy contracted by sailors on long voyages due to lack of vitamin C.

Vitamin C energizes the immune system to fight harder against cancer cells and other invading microbes.

For fruit sources, look to citrus such as oranges and pink grapefruit, kiwi fruit, berries of all kinds, and watermelon. The deep blue in blueberries and plums offers a clue that they're rich sources. In fact, blueberries are the most potent anti-oxidant that we can eat! Their cousins include red grapes, cranberries, cherries, prunes, and raisins.

The best vegetable sources include sweet red or green bell peppers, beets, broccoli, corn, eggplant, and avocados. Fruit and vegetable juices are also good sources, but beware of added sugars that increase calorie content such as high-fructose corn syrup, and added salt (high sodium).

The **B vitamins** are essential for normal functioning of the digestive system, to help convert carbohydrates into energy, to form red blood cells, to maintain the central nervous system, and for healthy brain, nerve, and skin cells. Sources include whole grains, lean meats and poultry, fish and shellfish, nuts, legumes (dried beans and peas, including soybeans), milk and other dairy products, green leafy veggies, eggs, potatoes, wheat bran, citrus fruits and juices, bananas, broccoli and its cousins in the cabbage family, and fortified complex carbohydrates in breads, pastas, and cereals.

The major function of **Vitamin D**, also known as the "sunshine vitamin," is to help the body absorb and maintain proper blood levels of calcium and phosphorus. In addition to ten to fifteen minutes of sunshine exposure without sunscreen three times per week, the best sources are dairy products, fish, and fortified cereals.

Vitamin E encourages reproduction of key infection-fighting cells called lymphocytes and boosts synthesis of antibodies. Good natural sources are whole grains, seeds, and vegetable oils. Oats are especially beneficial whole grains because they also contain valuable minerals. Cousins include wheat germ, flaxseed, whole wheat, barley, buckwheat. Many dieticians believe that it is impossible to get enough Vitamin E from dietary sources to fully protect against free radical damage, so recommend a daily supplement of 200-400 International Units (IU).

Vitamins are sensitive to light and heat in varying degrees, so store food away from light and refrigerate if it's fresh. To further conserve nutrients, cook with minimal amounts of water — and for a short time.

Carotenoids (think "carrots") increase lymphocytes and natural killer cells. Again, think color as you picture the best fruit and vegetable sources of these antioxidants: bright orange, red, green, and deep yellow. Choose fruits like cantaloupe, papaya, mango, and apricots. Choose vegetables like carrots, pumpkin, sweet potatoes, butternut squash, yams, red cabbage, tomatoes, spinach, kale, and other leafy greens.

Another potent *phytochemical* is found in soybeans. Sources of soy include tofu, soy powder, and soy-based vegetable protein. Other immune-strengthening compounds are found in garlic, onions, and the cruciferous vegetable family (broccoli, cauliflower, cabbage), as well as in aloe vera, algae, green tea, and a variety of other herbs.

Some fruits and vegetables also contain *flavonoids*, which are blood-thinning agents that offer the same heart-protective effects as red wine. Sources are celery, peppers, broccoli, grapes, lemons, garlic, and onions.

In addition to nutrients that we absorb, another reason to eat your fruits and veggies is that they also contain fiber (discussed later in this chapter). Your mother may have told you, "no fruit, no poop." It's still true!

Good news for chocolate lovers! Not only does dark chocolate taste wonderful, but studies show that just one serving provides antioxidants! Any kind works, but the darker the better, because the higher the cocoa content, the higher the antioxidant content. And, while chocolate is high in saturated fat, the kind it contains (stearic acid) doesn't seem to raise cholesterol levels. *Yes! Watch the calories, though.*

The same antioxidant family found in dark chocolate is also in red wine, grape juice, purple grapes, and green tea. So enjoy six ounces of juice/wine, 20 grapes, or two to three cups of green tea daily, too.

Combining these antioxidant fighters, especially Vitamins C and E, strengthens our immune systems better than any one alone. Eat several servings of fruits and vegetables at the same meal. Eat them often.

Minerals are essential to many bodily processes, from bone formation to functioning of the heart and digestive system. Since they are inorganic, minerals in foods are indestructible, but if food is boiled, discarded water carries nutrients down the drain — use only a small amount of water when cooking. Processed food also has fewer minerals. They are removed when grains are refined into flour.

Minerals are generally compounds with names that end in "ium," like calcium, magnesium, potassium, selenium, as well as iron and zinc, and trace amounts of others. Of these, sodium, calcium, and iron are of special concern in the typical American diet because, on average, we consume too much sodium and too little of the others. Not only does calcium build and maintain strong bones and teeth, but it also helps regulate heartbeat and other muscle contractions, is necessary for blood clotting, and may also prevent hypertension. If you take a medication for high blood pressure, increase your calcium intake from foods and take a supplement.

While iron deficiency is common in Americans (ads refer to "iron-poor blood"), the RDA (recommended daily requirement) is so small (15 mg) that a standard multivitamin can satisfy our needs, unless iron is depleted from

> Eat breakfast like a king, lunch like a prince, and dinner like a pauper.
> — Adelle Davis

strenuous activity or blood loss that causes anemia. The best sources of iron are red meats, so vegetarians are at some risk if they don't consume enough green leafy veggies, dried fruits, and legumes. If in doubt, ask a dietician.

How do I prevent more free radical damage?

Adopt a healthy lifestyle that helps your body destroy the *free radical* agents and restores balance to your body. Here's what you can do:

- Eat fruits, vegetables, and oily fish to zap those "rust" mongers with antioxidants.
- Take vitamin and mineral supplements.
- Avoid eating the empty calories that come from foods/drinks with little or no nutrient value — no junk food!
- Consume no more than 30% of total calories from fat and 10% from saturated fat. Avoid trans fat, if possible.
- Stop eating when you're full. Don't overeat!
- Stop smoking or don't start! Smoking greatly increases the concentration of free radicals in the blood.

Do I need to take supplements? Which ones?
Do you want to be all you can be? Fortifying food intake with vitamins and minerals is a good idea for us survivors. While our diets probably give us enough nutrients to prevent deficiencies, with all the rewiring demands on our bodies, we need more than the minimum. Nutritional supplements can help calm an overactive immune system, too. Because of possible interactions, though, consult with your physician about taking supplements — regardless of reported beneficial results. To help reduce the immune activity triggered by eating, take them about an hour before your biggest meal of the day, if possible.

Special survivor groups who especially need to take supplements include smokers, elderly people, daily soda/cola drinkers, and frequent aspirin takers. Why? Every cigarette kills 25 mg of vitamin C, older people often don't consume enough vitamin-rich foods, soda/cola interferes with mineral balance, and aspirin interferes with the metabolism of Vitamin C and some B vitamins. Another reason not to drink alcohol in excess: heavy consumption depletes both Vitamins B and C.

While smokers definitely need to replace the Vitamin C that each cigarette destroys, interactions with medications may increase their nutrient needs, too. If you smoke, talk with a dietician about this.

More reasons to supplement: water-soluble vitamins like B and C are especially vulnerable to changes in our body chemistry, Vitamin E stores are easier to maintain with supplementation than with food, and variations in fluid balance occur in natural monthly cycles, especially in females. Essential minerals, such as zinc and selenium, may or may not be provided by diet — depending on food selection!

Numerous experts recommend the following daily supplements: 1000 milligrams (mg) of Vitamin C divided into two doses, 1500 mg of calcium, up to 2000 IU of Vitamin D, 400 IU of Vitamin E (preferably natural d-alpha tocopherol), 25,000 IU of beta-carotene, 200 micrograms (mcg) of selenium, and a B vitamin that contains the RDAs of all the Bs. Adding Omega-3 (fish oil), a natural anti-inflammatory, ensures that your fish oil intake is adequate, especially if you aren't a regular fish eater.

Coenzyme Q_{10} in a daily dose of 100-200 mg has also recently been recommended by numerous health professionals as an antioxidant. It is one of the fuels that mitochondria, the power plants in each of our cells — including our brain cells — need to generate energy.

How to find what you need? For basic supplements, consider a packet of multiple pills. It is more cost-effective and easier than opening several bottles. You also avoid unbalancing your system with too much of one nutrient and not enough of another. A multiple vitamin-mineral pill with adequate amounts would be too big to swallow. Supplements need not be expensive, but do buy reputable brands to ensure that they meet standard United States Pharmaceutical (USP) requirements. Because the Food and Drug Administration (FDA) does not regulate supplements, some bottles may not contain what's listed on the label.

Attention: junk-food eaters! Vitamins work with other nutrients in food, so a supplement can't replace healthy eating and can't be a lazy person's path to good nutrition!

Are there special supplements to support our survivor-brains?
While you will no doubt hear about all the latest and greatest brain-boosters, **Ginkgo biloba** stands out. Used in Chinese medicine for thousands of years and in Germany for several decades, it is gaining attention in the US — particularly after respected medical journals documented that it helped to improve mental and motor performance in people with mild forms of dementia (Margen, 1992; Johnson, 1999).

Called a cerebro-active substance, Ginkgo's anti-clotting and antioxidant capabilities prevent degeneration of neurons and enhance blood flow and oxygen into the brain. The recommended dosage is 120-240 mg spread throughout a day. For a brain booster, the cost is reasonable, especially in large-sized bottles.

Healthful Eating Plans

To develop a healthful eating plan you choose foods that you like — and that also include the forty different nutrients you need. Regardless of how many calories you consume, most nutritionists recommend a diet that includes 45-60% carbohydrates, 20-30% protein (75-200 grams a day), and 20-30% fat (40-60 grams a day).

Fat is contained in most foods, so don't worry about consuming enough. In fact, most Americans eat 30-50% of their total calories in fats, especially if they eat a lot of fast food and processed foods. Regardless of total daily calories, dieticians recommend that you:

- Consume only 10% of your calories as saturated fat, which causes inflammation and raises your risk for heart disease.
- Avoid or consume only tiny amounts of trans fat, which lowers HDL (good cholesterol) and raises LDL (bad cholesterol).
- Consume no more than 300 mg of total cholesterol.
- Consume no more than 2400 mg of sodium, which increases blood pressure and can lead to stroke. *Do we need that?*
- Consume no more than 300 grams of total carbohydrate in a 2000-calorie diet or 375 grams in a 2500-calorie diet.
- Consume 25 grams of dietary fiber in a 2000-calorie diet and 30 grams in a 2500-calorie diet to improve digestive functioning.

Here's an example of a 2500-calorie diet plan:
Carbohydrates: 55% of 2500 =1375 calories.
Proteins: 25% of 2500=625 calories.
Fats: 20% of 2500=500 calories.

Personal experience. Years ago, out of curiosity, I checked the nutrient levels in my typical daily diet, rather than count calories. I found that I stayed well under 40 grams of fat per day and ate between 80-100 grams of protein (because I'm an athlete). I didn't count carbohydrates because overeating them wasn't a problem. Now, I don't count at all, usually only eat bread at lunch, rarely eat potatoes, and never eat junk food. If I begin to feel a little chubby, I check calories and reduce portion sizes, high-calorie snacks (such as nuts), and evening snacks of frozen yogurt or ice cream. To lose weight, I either don't replace my ice cream supply or eat from a bowl rather than eating from the carton — fun, but fattening!

Why do I need a plan/food budget? How do I start?

Like everything else post-injury, we need to optimize our eating to provide our brains and bodies with the nutrients needed to rewire. Remember our car-and-fuel analogy? After you check labels and read calorie charts for a while, you'll have a sense of typical nutrient amounts and won't need to continually watch and measure everything.

Food labels usually list the number of total calories and fat calories in a serving, and sometimes indicate amounts of fat from each source and percent of daily recommended amounts (RDA and % Daily Value).

To begin your study, it is helpful to know what you currently consume. Here are some steps to follow for a week:

- Weigh yourself once or twice a week, on the same days each week.
- List the ingredients and amounts of your favorite foods and drinks.
- Keep a food diary of what you eat, including the total number of calories in the amount you normally consume — *be honest!* To make it easier, maybe tape-record rather than write it.

Now, consider the results: if you want to feel better and/or lose or gain weight, change one thing at a time until you're satisfied. The first rule of any successful plan is no deprivation! Eat what you like — just less of it — and exercise more.

This is too confusing! Is there an easier way?

You can set up a personalized plan on your computer by going to www.MyPyramid.gov — the USDA site designed to help you plan and assess your food choices. Under "Subjects," choose "MyPyramidPlan," then input your age, height, weight, gender, and activity level. The site then suggests a total number of calories and amounts from each food group.

For example, for a 21-year-old male who is 6 feet tall, weighs 180 pounds, and is physically active for 30-60 minutes most days, the plan suggests 3000 calories. Of those calories, this man needs 10 ounces of grains, 4 cups of vegetables, 2.5 cups of fruits, 3 cups of milk, and 7 ounces of meats and beans. He can consume 10 teaspoons of oils and 520 calories worth of extra fats and sugars to stay at 180 pounds.

In contrast, a 35-year-old, 130-pound female, active for 30-60 minutes a day, needs only 2000 calories. Of those calories, she only needs six ounces of grains, 2.5 cups of vegetables, 2 cups of fruits, 3 cups of milk, and 5.5 ounces of meat and beans. She can consume six teaspoons of oils and needs to limit her extra fats and sugars to 265 calories to remain at her weight. If she increases her activity to more than 60 minutes a day, she can consume 2400 calories.

How do I understand nutritional labels?

You've no doubt seen these labels and maybe you have ignored them. A better idea is to use the information to ensure your diet is a healthy one because excess fat, sugar, and calories can sneak up on us if we're unaware of the nutrient content in the food that we like.

Basically, you want to choose foods that are low in saturated fats, trans fats, cholesterol, salt, and added sugar. Food makers are sneaky about adding unhealthy substances, so help yourself out by reading those labels! A clue to added sugar is any word that ends in "ose." For example, fruit sugar is fructose and milk sugar is lactose.

Start at the top with "serving size." Is the amount realistic? For example, one serving of ice cream is typically listed as ½ cup. Do you know anyone who eats only that amount? Likewise, a beverage serving is often listed as eight ounces, yet cans are often 12-ounce and most glasses at fast food places are far larger than that.

Next, check the number of servings in the package. Many contain more than one, which increases calories, nutrients, and percentage of Daily Value (DV), which is based on a 2,000-calorie diet and is a general guide. The DV can help you link nutrients in a serving to your total daily diet, showing if a particular food is high (20%) or low (5%) in a nutrient.

Now check the total fat, saturated and trans fat, cholesterol, and sodium, looking at percentage of Daily Value (DV). The total carbohydrate listing includes sugars, for which there isn't a DV, so limit added sugar, which adds calories but not other nutrients. Finally, check the number of grams of protein to ensure an adequate daily total amount. Although most Americans consume enough, athletes and growing bodies need about half their body weight in grams. Make sure your protein sources are healthy ones!

Nutrition Questions and Answers

How can I know what is the healthiest food to eat?

Remember to choose food with vibrant colors such as red, blue, yellow, orange, and green, bright like an artist's palate. Brown and white are okay for accent colors. Let's develop a plan to make this easier. If we plan — or think about — how to get the nutrients we need, we'll have a better chance of optimally fueling ourselves.

Just think energy in, energy out; garbage in, garbage out. To a large extent, how we fuel ourselves determines how we perform. Just remember how you felt the day after you ate large portions of something greasy and/or drank excessive amounts of alcohol.

What is the food-mood connection?

We know that food affects our moods: caffeine wakes us up, chocolate lifts our spirits, milk and cookies relax us, and a greasy pizza can dull our thinking and put us to sleep. How does this work? The natural chemicals in our food influence the production, interaction, and harmony of neurotransmitters, which in turn affect our moods.

Do you want to relax? Eat a protein food that contains tryptophan (such as milk products) with something that contains sugar (such as fruit or cookies). Our brains manufacture the calming neurotransmitter serotonin from this combination.

Do you need an energy pick-up in the late afternoon? Eat a complex carbohydrate, low fat, low protein snack. For example, enjoy whole grain crackers or a small bagel with nut butter and veggies or a piece of fruit with a handful of nuts or low-fat cheese, yogurt, or milk, or eat half an energy bar. Adding caffeine can stimulate you from one to seven hours. If you want only a little buzz, drink just a few sips. While coffee provides the most caffeine, black or green tea packs as much punch as Coke, Pepsi, Mountain Dew, or Sunkist soft drinks. Bottled juices vary in caffeine amounts and some decaf coffee isn't totally decaf. Experiment!

Do you want to be alert? Eat a protein food like turkey, fish, or cheese — with a slice of bread, whole grain crackers, or pretzels to provide carbohydrates so your body can manufacture the neurotransmitter dopamine.

Beware of the sugar merry-go-round that can occur if you eat a sugary snack on an empty stomach — especially with a caffeine beverage! Simple sugars are metabolized so fast that your energy first skyrockets and then it plummets. First, a sugar high, then a sugar low! You can avoid this rebound effect by eating a piece of fruit as a snack — the fiber slows the response — or eat sugary foods after a meal containing some protein and some fat to slow down the metabolizing process. Understanding the food-mood connection can help us balance our brains and behavior. To learn how different foods affect your moods, observe and then record your body's response to what and when you ate, and how you felt, at that time and later. You will begin to see what foods work best in your life and which ones to avoid.

How many times a day should I eat?
Whenever you're hungry, which is probably four to six times per day. The stomach empties about every four hours, so if we eat at least that often, we're usually not hungry — unless all we've consumed is quickly digested carbohydrates — sugars! For example, if we take a soda-and-candy-bar break, the immediate energy charge is followed by an energy drop. Thus, we need another refueling — leading to that familiar, and awful, energy rollercoaster.

Traditionally, Americans eat "three squares" a day. People of other nations eat more frequently, snacking between their meals. Besides reducing stress on our immune system, eating more than three times a day balances our blood sugar. It eliminates the mid-afternoon slump and the need to grab whatever we can find — usually unhealthy high fat/sugar foods — because we're too hungry to think about what we're doing. We also don't overeat at dinner because we're not so famished!

Those who are less active and burn fewer calories may feel better if they eat smaller meals more frequently, too.

How can I eat all day and not get fat?

If we eat foods that are low in fat and calories — like fruits, vegetables, and whole grains — we can eat many times a day, maintain a lean physique, and stay regular. The key here is "low in fat and sugar."

> Never eat more than you can lift.
> — *Miss Piggy's Guide to Life* as told to Henry Beard

Many studies show that if people maintain a stable (balanced) blood sugar, it helps them keep both their short-term and long-term goals. Short-term goals include eating foods that are the healthiest for us; long-term goals may include achieving a desirable weight or body size.

Personal experience. Besides water, I keep a supply of energy bars in my car to munch whenever I choose, which is always post-running and often mid-afternoon. Typically, I eat a few bites and then stash the rest in a baggie. At home, my favorite snacks are apple slices, almonds, and cherry tomatoes. If I'm really hungry and need energy before a workout, sometimes I'll dab peanut butter on apple slices. My bike bag always carries an emergency energy bar, too.

Why do I do this? To stay in control of my health and save money! If our blood sugar stays level, our brains work better, and we don't have to spend money needlessly on some fatty fast food. Plus — that control factor — we can eat what we choose and when we choose.

What is fiber, why do I need it, and where do I find it?

Fiber is an indigestible plant material that is needed for bowel regularity. Moving waste matter quickly and frequently is essential to overall health.

Because we can't digest it, fiber works like a natural laxative, stimulating our intestinal walls. Some kinds of fiber (such as that found in apples and oats) may even lower our circulating cholesterol to offer some protection against heart disease. Fiber also provides a bonus for weight watchers. Because it absorbs water, it makes us feel full after eating — think popcorn. Be sure to drink adequate water to smooth the passage!

When we eat, our food is broken down into usable and unusable fragments. What we don't need or can't digest is eliminated, along with old intestinal cells and good bacteria that live in our colon. Although we need these bacteria to help us break down our food, without fiber to eliminate them after they have finished their jobs, they start to ferment and produce gas and a certain odor. Fermenting, cancer-causing bacteria in waste also allows more time for invasion of sensitive colon membranes leading to discomfort and dysfunctions like constipation, hemorrhoids, diverticulosis (pouches in the bowl wall), and eventually to cancer.

Finding fiber is easy. Eat your fruits and veggies along with whole grains and beans. All plant foods provide fiber, so there is no reason to add commercial laxative products — especially if you exercise to help move your food along!

I'm not a big fan of vegetables. Can I drink juice instead?

How about if you do both? If you drink juices, beware of those with high sodium content — your daily limit is 2400 mg — and/or high calorie counts. Diluting juices with water helps to reduce these and lowers the price per serving. For even more nutritional punch, add a pinch of spices like turmeric and cumin, garlic, or ginger. To warm your body in the winter, heat the juice in a microwave. Accompanying your lunch with vegetable juice is healthy and may appeal to your taste buds!

Can comfort foods fit in my diet plan?

Yes — just be sure you're eating out of hunger for food, rather than another need. Are you feeling out of balance and scattered? Before you eat, ask yourself what kind of hunger you feel — food, sleep, exercise, sex? Then, satisfy that specific need. Maybe go back to your heart center with music. I know this sounds too easy, but if we're honest, we can save ourselves a lot of pain — and unwanted fat — if we respond to the real need. For example, if you need a hug, find a person or teddy bear or pillow and get it. Food only solves the hungry-for-food problem.

You know which comfort foods satisfy your own particular needs, but common ones include ice cream, bread, chips and dip, and sweets of various kinds, such as doughnuts. Chocolate in all sorts of divine concoctions is a favorite of many, especially of women who tend to prefer sweets. Men, on the other hand, tend to choose salty and protein foods. Eat a small amount and see if you're satisfied. If not, do something else.

Personal experience. When I grew up in Minnesota, everybody loved ice cream, which we ate frequently. Not a problem, then. Fast forward 40 years. Now, as an aging athlete with a lower metabolic rate, eating ice cream frequently means I get fat and jeopardize my sports performance. What to do? Eat non/low-fat or no-sugar-added yogurt or ice cream! But how much? Most labels list a serving as a half cup which, to me, is barely enough to feed a two-year old. So I add a drizzle of low-calorie chocolate syrup to a cup of my current favorite and I'm happy. Not only can I eat what I want, but I stay slim. Success!

Nobody likes to cook! Does convenience food fit in a healthy diet?
Yes, if you remember to first check fat, carbohydrate, and calorie contents before mindlessly eating. If these numbers are higher than your plan allows, you can still eat it with no guilt if you reduce your food intake for the next few days and/or increase your activity so the extra food does not add up to extra body fat. Generally, healthful eating means: low-fat meats or fish, sauces made with veggies or fruit, and large portions of whole (brown) grains and greens. Now, let's get specific:

Is Chinese food a favorite? Try shrimp and vegetable stir-fry with steamed rice. Most charts list this as 606 calories and 14 grams of fat. Maybe try chicken chow mein, vegetable lo mein, or stir-fried vegetables with chicken or meat. A veritable disaster, however, is a box of kung pao chicken with rice. The serving size is the problem, more than the food, since a box typically contains 1600 calories. Perhaps share the box with a friend or save half in your refrigerator for lunch tomorrow.

Like Italian food? Skip the cheesy lasagna. It's loaded with fat and is 1000 calories — or 1300 with a salad and high-fat dressing. Savor the flavors of veggies and tomato sauce with your choice of protein.

Is home-style your style? Skinless rotisserie turkey breast with new potatoes, steamed vegetables, and hot cinnamon apples only clocks in at 595 calories and nine grams of fat. Why? The fat is in the skin that we didn't eat! Other low-cal ideas include meat-loaf sandwich — no cheese, chicken soup with corn bread and zucchini, or white-meat chicken.

Mouth watering for Mexican? Skip the refried beans made with lard, the deep-fried (hard) taco shells, the enchiladas dripping with melted cheese and loaded with sour cream — providing enough fat and calories to last a week! Try a whole-wheat veggie burrito with black beans and rice for only 582 calories and nine grams of fat. If you skip — or go light on — the cheese and sour cream, other good choices include a soft taco with chicken, lettuce, tomatoes, salsa, rice, and whole beans or steak fajitas, light on the guacamole. Replace sour cream with plain yogurt — it's good!

Can I eat fast food in a healthy diet?

Yes, if you eat smart and keep your weekly food budget in mind. To include fast food in a healthy diet, check fat and calorie amounts in the foods you like. For example, pizza can be nutritious if you skip or reduce the greasy meat and cheese. If you need meat on it, ask for ham or Canadian bacon rather than pepperoni or sausage. Maybe try two slices of thin-crust or veggie pizza. In the following lists, notice that fat grams for some of the burgers exceed an entire day's allowance (40-60 grams)!

Restaurant	Food Item	Calories	total fat grams	sat fat grams
Burger King	Whopper	640	39	11
Burger King	Dbl Whopper W/Cheese	960	63	24
McDonald's	Big Mac	560	31	10
McDonald's	Qtr pounder w/cheese	530	30	13
Jack in the Box	Bacon/Ult/Cheesbrgr	1150	89	30
Hardee's	Monster Burger	970	67	29

Think you'll reduce calories and fat if you skip the beef? Sometimes yes, sometimes no:

Restaurant	Food Item	Calories	total fat grams	sat fat grams
Burger King	BK Broiler	550	29	6
Burger King	Chicken Sandwich	710	43	12
Mc Donald's	Chicken Fajita	190	7	3
Taco Bell	Chicken Club Burrito	540	31	10
Jack in the Box	Chicken Fajita Pita	280	9	4
Taco Bell	Chicken Fajita Wrap	460	21	6
Hardee's	Grilled Chix Sandwich	350	11	2
Wendy's	Grilled Chicken Sand.	310	8	2
Subway	Chick or Turkey Sub	320	5	1
KFC	BBQ Flav Chicken Sand.	260	8	1
Mc Donald's	Fish Filet Deluxe	510	20	5
Others	Tuna salad sand (w/mayo)	830	56	10
	Fried seafood combo	970	50	19
	Fried fish/shrimp (7/9 oz.)	520	26/24	10
	Broiled salmon	420	21	4
	Broiled low-fat fish	210	5	1

Think salads or veggies are always the best bet? Maybe.

Food Item		calories	total fat grams	sat fat grams
Mc Donald's	Grilled Chicken Salad (fat-free herb vinaigrette dressing)	170	2	0
Arby's	Roast Chicken Salad (reduced cal. ranch)	170	3	1
Taco Bell	Taco Salad w/salsa	840	52	15
Burger King	Broiled Chick. Salad (w/2 pkgs ranch)	560	48	12
Wendy's	Bacon/Cheese Potato	530	18	4
Arby's	Deluxe Baked Potato	740	36	16
Subway	Trky, Club, or Ham salad	160	3	1
Jack in the Box	Garden Chicken Salad (low-cal/Italian)	230	11	4

So — the bottom-line on fast food? It fits in a healthy diet if we eat other nutritious food. Just remember balance! Wear your "scientist hat." Skip high-fat meat, cheese, and dressings. Avoid fried food. Replace high carb foods with veggies. Share your meal, and enjoy the spices!

Do I need to eat with one hand on a calculator?

Only until you learn the approximate values of what you eat. For example, for about 100 calories you can eat either a piece of fruit, seven chips, a slice of bread, a potato, one-half cup of non-fat ice cream, or one tablespoon of butter, regular mayo, or salad dressing.

> We never repent of having eaten too little.
> — Thomas Jefferson

To markedly decrease calorie consumption for little taste difference, you might try low-fat salad dressing, margarine, and ice cream. No-sugar-added (NSA) ice cream is surprisingly delicious and creamy!

Is the portion size at restaurants a serving size?

Not on your life, unless you eat children's meals! Restaurant serving sizes often contain two to three times more food than nutrition guidelines consider a serving. *Picture a muffin — they're huge!*

Consider French fries: an official three-ounce serving of 1½ cups and 220 calories is equal to a McDonald's small fries! But McDonald's Super Size French Fries contains three cups, six ounces, and contributes 440 calories! Worse yet, most dinner-house restaurants serve even more fries — about 7 ounces!

Are you a pancake lover? An official serving is three pancakes: four ounces, 240 calories. A typical restaurant serving is four pancakes: 10 ounces, 610 calories — three times the fat, sodium, and calories — and not counting butter or syrup!

Do you like pasta? An official serving of one cup of spaghetti is 250 calories, including tomato sauce. A typical restaurant portion is 3½ cups and 850 calories, including sauce. Hmm — maybe choose again!

Thinking about guzzling a "Big Gulp"? Soft drinks can be tricky, too. To make it easier for us to compare beverages such as juices and milk, an official serving is eight ounces and 100 calories. But typical cans contain 12 ounces, which are 1½ cups and 150 calories. A 7-11

"Double Gulp" beverage contains 8 cups, 64 ounces, and 800 calories. Imagine empty calories taking up nearly half of one day's total calories! Since we're on fast food, let's talk about eating speed.

Is eating fast a problem? Does speed kill?
Yes, for several reasons, so put that fork down between bites! One, your brain takes 20 minutes to register if it's full or not. If you eat everything on your plate in five or ten minutes, you may eat more than you want, but it's too late! So, if you're full before your plate is clean, save the leftovers for the next time you're hungry. Doing this will save not only money, but also later food preparation.

And eating can be an enjoyable social experience. But if all you do is stuff your face, it's not very social, is it? Also, to enable our bodies to use nutrients, we need to chew the food into small enough pieces that our digestive enzymes can break it down. So, take a bite, put your fork down, and chew your food — your entire body will be happier.

Do you ever wonder why some restaurants play loud and fast music? We eat and drink a lot and then leave! How does your body respond? To see for yourself, observe how your eating speed responds to different kinds of music. Hint: to help you eat slowly, play slow and soft music.

If it's healthy food, can I eat all I want?
Sure, if it's vegetables. Otherwise, not all you want — what you need is a different issue. It doesn't really matter if it's healthy or not when it's more than we need. While it's true that our bodies respond better to

> One should eat to live, not live to eat.
> — Moliere

healthy food, when our "fuel tank" is full, it's full. Whether the food is of lesser or greater quality doesn't affect the size of our tank — it's still extra.

To store extra belongings, people sometimes rent storage space. But when we eat extra fuel, our bodies just expand their built-in storage tanks — and get fatter and fatter. *Do you point the nozzle at the back seat when your car's gas tank is full?*

What difference does it make? Eating is what I like to do!
It matters a lot if you want to be healthy. Do you like the current state of
your body? To occupy yourself, investigate other activities such as sports
or computers. Once you know the content of the food you eat, it can
become a game to keep you satisfied — maintaining the flavor of foods,
while cutting the number of calories, carbohydrates, and fat grams.

Initially, you may be somewhat surprised at the number of calories,
carbohydrates, and fat grams in the foods and beverages you like. For
example, one ounce of regular chips — about 12 chips — typically
contains 140-160 calories, 18 grams of total carbs, and 7-10 grams of fat
— a lot of carbs and fat if your daily budget is only 50 grams of each!
Plus, how many people eat only one ounce of chips?

How can I cut calories without reducing the flavor of my food?
For starters, eat smaller portions of your
favorites or eat half of a favorite bar or
treat and save the rest for a later time. *Just
a taste really can satisfy!*

For other ways, again think like a
scientist. Make a change and see if you
like it. If not, choose again. *To remember,
record what you do.*

For example, if you like regular milk
products, try the low-fat version. If that

> Eating everything you want is not that much fun. When you live a life with no boundaries, there's less joy. If you can eat anything you want to, what's the fun in eating anything you want to?
> — Tom Hanks

tastes okay, try the non-fat version. If you don't like it, stay with low fat
or mix whole milk and non-fat or add powdered non-fat milk to liquid
non-fat milk. Same with ice cream — try the reduced or no-sugar-added
versions.

How is the rate at which I burn calories established?
Metabolic rate is the speed our bodies burn fuel or calories. If we're
inactive, our rate is slow because our bodies don't need a lot of fuel just
to maintain basic functions like breathing.

As we age, our metabolic rates naturally decrease about one-half to
one percent every year over age 30. However, this rate of loss of lean
tissue — muscle and bone — occurs only if we don't intervene in the

process by exercising. If we strength-train twice a week and participate in activities such as walking, wheeling, cycling, etc. at a moderate pace for 30-60 minutes every day, we slow down the decrease. See Chapter 10 for activity tips.

How can I increase my metabolic rate?
While you cannot affect your gender or age, you can boost your body's rate of burning fuel in several ways:
- Strength-train. This increases lean muscle mass, which burns more calories and raises the amount of fuel your body needs.
- Do physical activities to use energy and increase lean muscle mass.
- Eat more often. It takes energy to burn your fuel, raising your metabolic rate about 5%! Just make sure to eat the same number of total calories per day or you'll gain weight.

How does lean muscle mass differ from fat?
Muscle is active tissue — meaning it takes energy (fuel) to stay alive. The more muscle we carry, the higher our basal metabolic rate is. Fat, on the other hand, is mostly inactive tissue.

Think about how children, adolescents, and athletes of all ages seem to eat all the time. They need to refuel their bodies frequently because they're growing, the percentage of muscle in their bodies is high, and their activities use a lot of energy.

When we don't use our muscles, they atrophy and lose tissue mass. Contrary to what some people may think, muscles don't turn to fat — they can't change composition. But they lose tone when they're not used, so they may look like fat. Muscle tissue is also denser and weighs more than fat tissue, so people with more muscle mass can weigh more and yet look leaner than fatter people. The percentage of body fat also increases with inactivity, so it's lower in more active people.

How many calories do I really need?
Consider how much energy you use for daily activities beyond basic bodily functions. If someone drives to work, sits at a desk, then sits in front of a TV in the evening, this sedentary person uses fewer calories than someone who is physically active for part of the day. What happens

if he fuels himself with more than his body needs that day? It's stored —
as fat — to be used when he's short of fuel on another day — or not! If
the fuel is not used, it's simply stored. And stored!

As you can see on www.MyPyramind.gov ("MyPyramidPlan")
eating is based on activity as well as age. Sedentary people may want to
try 1600-1800 calories per day. If you are very active, you may want to
consume around 3000 calories, and see what happens. For those in
between, experiment with a range of 1800-2800 calories. The body at
rest only uses about 50-60 calories per hour. So, if you want to eat that
cookie, get off the couch!

How can I prevent overeating?
We really can train our brains to like what we eat. For example, if large
amounts of sweets aren't eaten every day, the body and brain learns to
like fruits just as well. Treats can be eaten occasionally or in small
amounts daily. If a weekend brings a splurge, no big deal — just reduce
food intake for the next week and/or increase daily exercise to burn off
the extra calories.
- Eat only when hungry.
- Eat several (four to six) small meals a day, under 500 calories each.
- Eat early in the day when you're more active.
- Eat slowly.
- Stay hydrated with water or herbal beverages without caffeine.
- Exercise daily for at least 30 minutes.

I can't stop eating! What's going on? What can I do?
Several things can create this state:
- You may just be thirsty and not hungry. Drink a beverage and see if
  this helps.
- People may eat because they're bored or depressed. Distract your
  brain with activity. Are you still hungry?
- Eating serves as a source of comfort for some people. Maybe you're
  hungry for love, rather than food. See if socializing helps.
- Maybe you have a need for a nutrient that your body lacks. For
  example, if you crave ice cream, maybe you need more calcium.
  Milk is the best source. Determine how much you consume. If under

1500 mg daily from supplements and milk products, increase the amount. If your intake is adequate, perhaps your calcium pills are not properly absorbed. One way to test absorption is to drop the pill in a cup of vinegar. If it dissolves, it will also dissolve in your stomach. If not, buy a different brand.

- Another craving culprit may be a chemical like that found in diet drinks. Did you know that sugar substitutes may create a physical craving and actually cause you to eat more? Try it and watch yourself: When you're not hungry — after a meal, drink a diet soda and see if you don't search for something to eat! It's not hunger talking, it's the chemical. So eat a snack with a diet drink or don't drink them.

- Perhaps your physical need or "addiction" is actually food intolerance in disguise. You probably know which foods trigger you to eat non-stop. In that case, the particular food is the opposite of what you need. Try this approach: eat a small amount of the problem food a few times a week. Wear your scientist hat, observe what happens, and then explore your ideas with a nutritionist.

- If none of these ideas solve the problem, perhaps you're a non-taster, which is a physical — not psychological — problem. It means that your body doesn't register that you're satisfied because you haven't tasted anything, so you eat a lot in an attempt to taste.

- If none of these solutions work, the brain injury and/or medication may be the culprits again, so ask your health professionals for help.

Even if you're not a non-taster, add some spice to your life! In addition to enhancing taste, spices offer many other benefits. Some spices, like onions, garlic, allspice, and oregano stop the growth of food-borne bacteria. Capsaicin, the hot part of chilies, cools bodies by making them sweat! Other hot spices can trick you into thinking you've eaten more than you actually have, which is a bonus for dieters. Spices stimulate your senses, increasing your feeling of satisfaction after eating.

Personal experience. *My body is somewhat intolerant of corn. If, in the course of my day I eat corn in several forms (breakfast cereal and corn chips), I may find myself unable to stop eating the chips. This is due, in fact, to my eating more corn products over a few days than my body* *can digest well. So, I simply follow the SAFER plan — Stop, Assess, Fix, Examine, Retry — and stop the corn.*

Why do sugar cravings occur? How are sugar addictions treated?
You will be glad to know that it's really not a matter of weak will. Rather, some folks may be born to be sugar sensitive.

Studies that link sugar cravings to lowered levels of the neurotransmitters serotonin, dopamine, and beta-endorphin suggest that this addiction is similar to alcoholism and that it is inherited. In these individuals, food with high sugar content can be addictive, just like alcohol is for an alcoholic. The euphoric feelings that accompany eating sugar compel these highly sensitive people. Additionally, these high-sugar foods can act like opiates in our bodies and decrease our ability to feel pain — which is another reason they can be addictive.

Studies of families with several alcoholic members show that many are also addicted to sugar, and that those who crave sugar, alcohol, or both are responding to an imbalance in their neurotransmitters — thus, placing the blame on the condition and not the person.

If you suspect a sugar addiction: first try eating your sugar with something to slow down its absorption — like a little bit of protein and fat. Nuts work well. If that doesn't work, observe the effects of different foods on your moods. Then, with that information, seek professional help to help you balance your sensitive brain chemicals. Successful treatment approaches include medication, acupuncture, balanced nutrition, exercise, and increased exposure to light sources.

Is chocolate good for us?
Yes, but not if you eat too much. The theobromine, caffeine, and antioxidants are all good for you. High levels of fat and sugar make it a mixed blessing.

A chocolate bar that weighs 1.5 ounces contains 205 mg of phenolics, which improve the health of the circulatory system. Chocolate needs to be high quality — made from cocoa butter, not palm or coconut oil, to be healthful. And, the darker it is, the more phenolics it contains. Eat a little but make sure it fits in your food plan.

What about caffeine?

Want a quick no-calorie boost? Coffee and cola lovers know how to energize: drink caffeine. It stimulates mental and physical performance, improves mood, fights fatigue, speeds calorie burning, extends our ability to exercise or perform arduous physical tasks, and increases the power of painkillers.

The downside to caffeine is that, just like a lot of things, when the balance is disturbed, too much creates problems. Excess amounts can overstimulate the nerves to raise blood pressure, speed heartbeat, and promote heartburn, frequent urination, and/or diarrhea. These speed effects can lead to jitteriness, shakiness, irritability, and insomnia. Caffeine also interferes with the sedative effects of some medications, accentuates the effects of others such as oral decongestants, and triggers headaches with abrupt withdrawal.

To calm any concern about raising blood cholesterol levels, research shows that only certain brewing methods, like boiling and espresso, create this hazard. So, be moderate, caffeine-lovers, and be sure to get the okay of your physician.

Why do I need to drink a lot of water?

All our bodily functions and biochemical reactions require water to operate efficiently. We need water to digest food, remove waste products from our bodies, send electrical messages, regulate body temperature, lubricate our joints, and even to keep saliva moist in our mouths to prevent cavities and gum deterioration. If we don't hydrate properly, our cells dry out. Picture tanned leather! Drinking water also aids fat metabolism and helps decrease our appetites because we feel full longer.

To maintain fluid balance, we need to replace the water our bodies use every day. How much is that? Our bodies use about 50-100 ounces (six to 12 cups) every day. Divide your body weight in half for an approximate amount in ounces. You don't have to drink that much water, though. The liquid in other drinks (except alcoholic ones) also counts. So do the liquids in your foods, such as the juice in your apples or tomatoes.

Sleep

We need sleep to live. It's nutrition for our mind much like food is nutrition for our body. If we're deprived, we die — it's as simple as that. While some folks consider doing without sleep worthy of praise, in fact, it's more worthy of a dunce cap! If deprived of sleep, the brain's energy supplies run down. When this occurs, alertness, mood, and judgment decrease, which compromises our performance, safety — and happiness!

Sleep not only restores body and brain energy that is used for daily activities, but it also provides needed time for our brains to review the day's activities and store or discard information. The downtime of REM (Rapid Eye Movement) dreaming, which occurs with deep sleep, allows our brains to defrag — to use a computer term. And learning improves if it is immediately followed by restorative sleep — a good thing for us!

Sleep also balances the blood levels of the hormones that keep us healthy. During sleep, two hormones that we need to grow and to fight disease are increased and one (cortisol, released by the adrenal gland in response to stress) is decreased. However, if the brain is forced to stay awake, cortisol increases. High levels of it cause shrinkage in the hippocampus, the region of the brain that is responsible for learning and memory (Kotulak, 1998). *Like we need that!*

Ever feel run down from lack of sleep and then find yourself sick? It's not coincidence. Irrefutable evidence shows that getting enough sleep is vital to a healthy immune system and that accumulating sleep debt further compromises our systems. Even one night of partial sleep loss causes a significant decline in immune capabilities. And while a night of recovery sleep returns natural killer cells to their original strength the next day, other immune responses stay suppressed beyond one day.

To decrease your chances of a heart attack or stroke, sleep eight hours or more per night so that the hormones that increase right before awakening during REM sleep don't stress your heart and increase blood pressure (Friedman School, 2004).

Why else do we need enough sleep?

Is weight gain a problem? Perhaps you need more sleep. Studies find that a lack of sleep decreases leptin, a hormone that suppresses appetite and provokes a craving for starchy, sweet, high-carb foods. Lack of sleep can also lead to overeating to compensate for the loss of body heat, which can even become a chronic condition so that more food is needed to keep the body at its new setting.

Want to decrease your risk of diabetes? Get your Zs! Research shows inadequate sleep causes abnormal insulin and blood sugar levels — pre-diabetic conditions. This insulin resistance also may cause brain inflammation, a key process in the development of Alzheimer's (Roan, 2008). *Like we need more brain damage!*

Want to be decades older than you are? Sleep seven hours or less! Some lab blood tests of sleep-deprived men ages 27-42 looked more like those in their 60s. Despite the common misperception, recommended sleep amounts do not decrease as with age (Friedman School, 2004).

How much sleep do I need?

Sleep researchers suggest one hour of sleep for every two hours of wakefulness. Children, adolescents, and brain-injury survivors need more. Stabilizing our vital serotonin levels requires adequate sleep, so aim for between 8-10 hours per night. Your sleep is right if it refreshes you. Observe how you feel. Do you feel rested and able to cope with life's demands — and even have a little extra in your battery? Is your appetite under control? How's your mood?

What is good sleep hygiene?

To insure the deep restorative sleep necessary for optimal performance, sleep experts offer several suggestions (Scripps, 1989; Kotulak, 1998; Friedman School, 2004):

Daytime and evening tasks.
- Maintain regular arising hours. Brains and bodies like a routine.
- Expose yourself to bright light or sunlight shortly after you awaken to help set your biological clock.
- Participate in mental and physical activity — essential for balance and proper fatigue.
- Complete vigorous exercise at least three hours before going to bed.

- Avoid sleeping late or daytime naps lasting more than 20 minutes unless you're ill or fighting illness.
- Don't smoke. Nicotine stimulates and may cause a withdrawal wake-up.
- Spend some time every day with Nature, even just a few minutes.
- Manage stress with exercise, meditation, nature, diet, friends.
- Avoid drinking alcohol and caffeinated beverages late in the evening.
- Eat a light dinner between 5:30 PM and 7:00 PM to avoid excess stomach acid. Digestion raises metabolic rate and slows later in the day.
- Keep lights low near bedtime to prepare body and brain for sleep.

Nighttime tasks.
- Maintain a regular bedtime, even on weekends and holidays.
- Enjoy a small snack if hungry. Low blood sugar can cause agitation.
- Avoid stimulating activities, people, food, and drink. No alcohol!
- Relax with light reading, soft music, or a warm bath.
- Keep bedroom cool, quiet, inviting, and dark. Explore using the white noise of a fan to quiet body and mind.
- Use bedroom for sleep and sex only — not as an office or TV room.
- Go to bed as soon as you feel sleepy. Fighting it energizes you!
- To create a peaceful mind, try focusing on a sleep mantra — an image, thought, emotion, or memory — to help clear your mind.
- If your body is restless, get up, read, drink warm milk or herb tea, such as chamomile or peppermint. Return to bed when sleepy.
- If your mind is active, stay in bed! Lying motionless can be restful, too. Do relaxation exercises or visualize a peaceful scene.
- If sleepless after 20 minutes or so, get up. Read or make a to-do list for the next day. Making a plan relieves anxious thoughts.
- If you awaken, recite a mantra, breathe deeply, practice relaxation exercises, fantasize, or think other pleasant thoughts.

Is insomnia a problem?
To self-cure, first practice SAFER (Stop, Assess, Fix, Examine, Retry). Keep a log of activity, food, and sleep. Then correct obvious problems. If it continues, discuss the use of sleep aids — herbs, valerian, L-

tryptophan, melatonin, or prescription medications — with your health care team. Current medications, pain, indigestion, depression, anxiety etc. can all prevent restful sleep.

Summary

To nurture "my body, my car":

- Think artist's-palate colors when you choose foods.
- Eat slowly.
- Eat lots of brain food: fish, fruits, and veggies.
- Avoid junk food.
- Eat only when hungry.
- Maintain regular arising and sleeping hours.
- Avoid stimulating activities, people, food, or drink late in evening.

> You are what you eat.
> — Adelle Davis

Here's to smart brains, healthy bodies, and sweet dreams!

10
Physical Rewiring:
Healing Our Bodies, Ourselves

A brave heart is a powerful weapon.
— Rudy Garcia, triathlete & double amputee

Just do it! Play to create new brain cells! Discover the benefits of exercise and how physical activity helps you to rewire. This chapter describes what you need to get off the couch and get active so you can enjoy life again. To give your brain what it needs to motivate your body, we explore the latest research studies that show how exercisers far surpass those who don't — in every area of life.

We discuss the typical physical problems that we face and places that offer help. We explore ways to regain lost or damaged physical skills, including using an electrical muscle-stimulating device and mind-expanding movement therapy to increase the use of a damaged limb.

Answers to "What do I do when my body says go, but my head says no?" and other common exercise questions are here. Components of a fitness program are described, including how to set goals, choose exercise equipment and select activities.

To hopefully inspire you, my personal physical recovery journey is included. In the self-care section, you learn how to listen to your body and use pressure-point therapy and simple massage techniques on yourself. To know how many minutes of activity are needed to work off your favorite foods, see the list at the end of this chapter. Included are:

- Exercise benefits.
- Basics of an exercise program.
- Components of an exercise program.
- Exercise equipment ideas.
- Facilities and resources.
- Social and health benefits.
- Exercise questions and answers.
- Activity suggestions.
- Self-care.

Introduction

"Physical recovery — you're kidding! Heal my body myself? I don't think so. It's so damaged there's nothing left to mend. No can do."

> There are two ways you can go. You can continue life and keep going or you can go home and vegetate.
> — Don Hyslop
> (wheelchair racer)

Yes, you can! Explore how you can recover before you decide that you can't! Give it a go before you say no.

"You mean exercise? That's too much work. I get all I need by lifting a cold one. Anyway, I don't want to be an athlete or look like a movie star. I just want to feel better about myself and enjoy life again."

Okay — that can happen. What have you got to lose besides fat, poor muscle tone, inactive limbs, and that tired feeling? By the way, got anger? How's your self-esteem?

How good can you get? Nobody knows. Just Do It! See for yourself, because you can recover function.

"I don't think it'll work for me. My injury happened a long time ago and I stopped exercising when physical therapy ended."

Yes, it can still work! Studies show that everyone benefits — even those who haven't exercised for several years or whose injuries were long ago. Survivors can regain lost skills once they start to exercise again (Bray et al., 1987; Dordel, 1989).

"Maybe, but my injury was really bad. My arm (or leg) doesn't work right."

Remember the phrase "Use it or lose it"? Let's rephrase that: use it to lose it! — Lose what? Disability!

"Oh sure," you may think. "Fat chance I can't be disabled! Show me how that can happen."

OK — how about less disabled? Active folks feel better, act smarter, and can do more! Survivors who exercise are not only more mobile and productive — thus, more involved in their communities — but also happier and generally feel better (Gordon et al., 1998). Do you want a fitter body to act as a "chick (or guy) magnet"? How'd you like to boost your brainpower? How about greater control — of health, emotions, energy — everything in life? Active people with disabilities improve stamina, joint flexibility, muscle strength, and mood! (Surgeon General, 1996).

Still not convinced? "Many people with disabilities develop medical conditions due to lack of exercise" (Durstine, 2000). An inactive lifestyle decreases your cardiorespiratory (heart-lung) fitness. Less blood circulation to lower extremities can lead to osteoporosis (fragile bones), which can result in more dependence on others, less social interaction, and more disability!

Avoid the robot syndrome! Exercise prevents the kinds of problems that plague survivors who vegetate after discharge: weight gain, boredom, inactivity, depression, and fear of attempting challenging motor activities (Mercer & Boch, 1983).

So, if you want to feel, look, remember, and sleep better, fight off germs, move easier, and perform more activities — with greater energy, Just do it! *Okay, I believe that exercise can cure almost anything.*

Personal experience. *I remember when a twenty-something guy called me "one hot momma" one weekend and a different guy labeled me "a trophy" the next weekend! Who, me, at fifty-two years of age? How did this occur? Because I didn't believe the "it's not gonna happen" prognosis, I didn't believe the "you won't be able to..." prediction, and I didn't believe the "you can't do... anymore" statements.*

Exercise Benefits

Just for a moment, forget that activity is fun and movement brings joy — focus on health. Exercise can prevent and treat disease. By stimulating blood flow and tissue growth in muscle and bone, physical activity positively affects all bodily systems — whether disabled or not. Consider this research — and then get active (Gordon et al., 1998).

> The game of life is a lot like football. You have to tackle your problems, block your fears, and score your points when you get the opportunity.
> — Lewis Grizzard

Study of TBI Survivors

To explore the benefits of exercise for survivors, 240 individuals from various communities completed "Quality of Life and Health Interviews." The nearly 70% male participants were injured, on the average, about 10 years earlier. Of these, 27% exercised and 73% didn't.

In the preceding six months, exercisers swam, jogged, or bicycled for an average of thirty minutes per session, three times a week — definitely not a rigorous training schedule! While some of the differences between exercisers and non-exercisers were sharper than expected, one finding was a surprise: exercisers had sustained more severe brain injuries, as measured by loss of consciousness. Imagine that! Here are the results:

Overall health. Non-exercisers reported symptoms from their injuries significantly more frequently than exercisers, including nearly 35% who found it difficult to handle personal care versus 8% of the exercisers.

Improved physical health. Forty percent of the non-exercisers reported blurred vision compared to 14% of exercisers; similar numbers were found for waking up and staying awake. Exercisers were more mobile and independent.

Improved cognitive skills. Does regular activity make us smarter? Not exactly, but it helps us to function better. Far fewer exercisers than non-exercisers reported problems learning, remembering, following directions, organizing, using their time, planning, caring for themselves and others, and even seeing others' points of view.

Improved emotional health. Want to be happier? Fewer exercisers reported feeling depressed (12.5%) than non-exercisers (33.7%). Irritability and nervousness was reported for 60% of the sedentary folks versus 40% of the active ones. Boredom was a problem for more than twice as many couch potatoes as those who exercised.

Increased productivity and community involvement. Exercisers not only felt less impaired, they were more mobile and productive. Integrating better into the community means more opportunities to socialize and meet others of the opposite sex!

Unimportant Factors for Exercise Participants

Time since injury or activity is unimportant. Some improvement in functional physical activities can occur long after injury and initial rehabilitation, even if your underlying neuromotor abilities remain unchanged. You still may regain lost skills — once you start therapy again (Bray et al., 1987; Dordel, 1989).

> Movement and the functioning of the brain are eminently connected.
> — Rick Rogers

Physical disability is not a deterrent. Paralyzed? Use a wheelchair? These factors are not obstacles to activity or being productive. Research shows that motor disability does not have a significant impact on rehabilitation or long-term disability (Cohadon et al., 1988).

How can I exercise with spastic muscles?

First, consider if the spasticity prevents or reduces your ability to do something.

If it does, explore ways to reduce the spasticity, in consultation with your health professionals, of course. In addition to medication, some effective methods include using ice, electrical stimulation, muscle vibration, various relaxation techniques, and stretching, both manually and with pulleys. Splints, casts, braces, and other kinds of orthotic devices may also manage spastic muscles. Magnet therapy is certainly worth a try, as discussed in Chapter 8.

In most cases, using a physical modality such as ice, exercise, and/or orthotic devices combined with an anti-spasmodic medication can reduce spasticity to a manageable state (Griffith, 1983).

How Exercise Delivers Benefits

What happens when we exercise our cardiovascular system?
Activity that raises heart rate also increases oxygen flow to the brain through blood. Exercise stresses and strengthens the heart, increasing the heart's stroke volume, so that the heart pumps more fresh blood through the body and to the brain each time it beats.

How can exercise improve cognitive skills such as memory?
When we power up our furnaces, not only do our neurons receive more nutrients — exercise improves our oxygen consumption, so we get more out of every breath! More efficient use of oxygen can improve our thinking. Here's why: while the brain comprises just 2% of our body weight, it receives 15% of the blood, consumes 15% of the oxygen and 70% of its glucose (blood sugar), which gives us our energy. Physical activity also develops more capillaries around neurons and may help to produce growth factors that are related to improved cognitive function.

What kinds of activities deliver these benefits?
Any rhythmic movement, indoors or outdoors, that continues for at least ten minutes at a time brings benefits. Naturally, the longer the activity and the more body parts that are involved, the greater the gains to your body, like swinging your arms while walking.

> You keep on getting what you're getting when you keep on doing what you're doing.
> — Anonymous

Weight training — especially the nonstop variety called circuit training — elevates heart rate too, but not as much as cardiovascular activities do. Keep reading for activity ideas.

How vigorous and how much physical activity?
If the thought of a hardcore workout turns you off, here's great news! To achieve health benefits, activity doesn't need to be strenuous and can be done in several short sessions. Experts currently recommend 30-60 minutes of moderate activity every day, which can be done in 10-minute sessions if that works best for you. "Moderate" means exercising hard enough to break a sweat, yet talking without gasping for breath.

Health benefits seem to be proportional to amount of activity. The more you do, the more you benefit — and everything counts — including activities like cleaning and yard work! So how hard can it be to incorporate fun and varied activities into your lifestyle?

What won't exercise do?
Although I happen to believe that exercise is the answer for just about everything, it cannot work a miracle to eliminate all pain and disability. Nothing changes the fact of the disability. However, physical activity can change how the disability affects you by reducing the handicapping effects of brain injury that a sedentary lifestyle worsens, such as reduced mobility, flexibility, strength, and depressed mood!

How do I start my physical rewiring?
Seek referrals to physical therapists who specialize in your interest areas. Request programs that you can do and ask them to show you what equipment to use — and to avoid — and how to adapt generic

> You're never a loser
> until you quit trying.
> — Mike Ditka

equipment. Ask about programs and audio/video tapes that you might like. Find a group or class you can join. Then to avoid the robot syndrome — just do it!

Basics of an Exercise Program

After reading about how exercise improved the lives of other survivors, you've decided you want to be healthier, fitter, stronger, smarter, and happier, too. Good. Now let's plan how to get where you want to go.

Goals

Decide what you want to achieve and when. Be realistic; make an adjustable timeline. If you are currently inactive, start with 10 minutes every day — or twice a day — for a week. If this feels good, add a few minutes every day. If that's too easy, increase it more. Listen to your body. Tell health care professionals about your goals. Ask about any limitations, medication effects, and warning signs of overexertion.

What kinds of goals should I set?

Beyond enjoying activity, most likely your primary goal is to "improve my health." This means developing and improving strength, flexibility, and endurance, which are all vital for a healthy functioning body. Want quick results? Strength training helps to develop the muscular power you need to do cardiovascular (endurance) activities, which is key for improving heart and lung efficiency and is the best way to reduce body fat. Stretching keeps your muscles supple and improves range of motion. We survivors likely need to add "develop and improve balance" to our goal list.

To "improve appearance" may be a secondary goal. To look better means gaining muscle and losing fat. Our bodies lose about a half pound of muscle every year starting in our mid-twenties, but strength training counteracts this natural phenomenon. And muscle is more active than fat — one pound of muscle burns about 35 calories a day but fat burns only two!

Another goal may be to participate in athletic events. These are wonderful places to meet others who like to do what you do. Join outdoor events such as walks/runs, cycling/wheeling, water contests, and triathlons (swim-bike-run). Indoor events invite us to dance, fence, do martial arts, or enter bodybuilding contests. Set goals that are achievable so you can be proud of your achievements. You can do it!

Locate resources. Because knowledge is power, arm yourself with information. Contact local facilities. Ask about their programs, fees, and if financial help is offered. Buy or borrow fitness books and/or videos. *Weight Training for Dummies* and *Fitness for Dummies* books are fun to read and helpful. See Resources for good web sites.

Motivation

Okay, you set your goals and gathered your resources. Next, ask yourself what it will take to actually get you to do what you resolved. For most of us to be active, we need to enjoy what we do, feel good about it, and do it well — or we won't do it. How can we enjoy exercise? Make it fun to do — and achievable.

Key factors: Select a high-energy time, choose tunes you like, wear clothes you feel good in, go where you want to go, do what you want to do with people you like — or alone. Take your ID with you. All of these things are within your control. If something doesn't feel right, choose again!

How do I handle obstacles?

"What do I do when my body says 'go!' but my head says 'no!'?" If you've set goals and made time for it, other issues may obstruct you.

> Play is the answer — the answer to the unsuccessful fitness program, the answer to the unsuccessful life." Once you've found your play, all else will be given to you.
> — George Sheehan

What if I just don't feel like exercising?

Do it anyway! Start with some positive self-talk — "I know it'll feel good." Then promise yourself that you can stop if, after ten minutes, you still don't want to do it. By that time, "I'm already ten minutes into it, so I may as well keep going!"

Another strategy is to tell yourself that you're not exercising, you're just getting outdoors to investigate — the latest flowers, animals, cars, businesses, etc.; meet new people; socialize with your neighbors; play; or go to the mall to just start walking and window shopping.

Try a different activity and/or setting. Sometimes we think we don't want to exercise when we just need to find the right activity! Do your ten minutes. Then, if both body and brain rebel and want to quit, stop what you're doing and try something else. Maybe do a less demanding activity such as yoga or stretching. Maybe even do work — but keep those good vibes coming. Any kind of change will help. Be your own coach.

Yet another idea is to not think about it. Just put your shoes on and go outside — you'll think of something fun to do! Remember how, as children, we always wanted to go play? How easy it was to entertain ourselves! Rediscover that child in you again.

Other physical needs. Start exercising and do 10 minutes. If neither body nor mind wants to go on, stop and ask yourself, "If it's not different exercise, do I need food or sleep?" Perhaps your body is hungry or tired and that's why it doesn't want to go. You may need to try all three options before you find the right answer. Eventually, you'll learn your "stop" signs and know what to do right away.

Boredom. If boredom hits in the middle of an activity, change the pace. As hard as it is to believe, even when you think you're tired, increasing the speed is possible! After fifty feet of blazing speed, the previous pace may not be boring anymore! Slowing down is another option.

Discouragement with learning new skills. Initial frustration often accompanies trying something new. Overcoming this may involve learning to like your new activity or sport. Just Do It! — that works here too, because "behavior change precedes attitude change" — as my therapist, Mary Alice Isenhart, proclaimed one day in 1992 when I said I didn't feel like doing something. So, do the activity — you may begin to like it.

Personal experience. Some of us need to convince ourselves that our attitude will indeed change before we do something. Here's how it worked for me: after hating running for years, I told myself, "You will like running." I knew that to be good at something, I had to like it and I needed to run to do triathlons. It worked! I began to like to run, ceased being embarrassed about my lack of speed and big legs, and — I got faster!

The success of this approach depends on more than just drive — we must also know what we need to enjoy something. For me, it's a scenic and peaceful location. So I mostly run on the beach at low tide and often finish with a refreshing ocean dip, which assures a joyful experience! That way, if my run is less than spectacular, the ocean will make it all better. When the tides don't cooperate, I run in the riverbed or local park.

If it rains or the time is short, I hop on the stair-stepper on my porch and enjoy the scenery of the neighborhood! Nothing stops me!

Staying motivated. Like other important events, write your exercise schedule on your calendar or date book. Record your progress in a fitness notebook. Include progress notes like medical professionals do — for example, "can wheel a block without tiring" or "can lift arm to comb hair." Reward efforts, time spent, and progress. This doesn't mean what you tried but what you did! Select non-food rewards — outings, video time, etc. Use photos to keep you inspired! Post photos of other bodies you like and your own developing one to keep you on track.

Bottom line. Just like anything else, just do it! Take that first step. Walk or roll a block or two, then five — maybe a mile after a few weeks. Finish the first ten minutes of a program and keep going because it feels good. Push out eight — and then ten — repetitions with weights. What happens? You smile and hopefully hear some positive self-talk: "I did it! It wasn't that hard and it was kind of fun! Maybe I can do other things, too."

Components of an Exercise Program

Balance and movement

Moving requires spatial awareness and balance. So in order to get in gear, we need to know where we are in space. Before our injuries, we naturally self-corrected — now, our bodies need to relearn to balance.

Remember the telephone story? Our wires are down and, because the information flow from our various *proprioceptors* (balance sensors) is not received, sent, or interpreted correctly, our feet can't talk to our brains — coordinated movement isn't possible. We're all born with millions of different kinds of balance sensors in the muscles, tendons, ligaments, and joint capsules of our bodies. Our body parts need to relearn how to communicate with one another.

Physical therapists use special methods to rewire the circuits that you need to move. Some of the activities to reeducate limb coordination may seem

> Movement develops intelligence.
> — Rick Rogers

childish — do them anyway! You will likely play some fun games, too. Keep trying different methods and you will improve!

Do any programs focus on movement education?
Yes, specialized programs can teach you how to move better. You've probably heard of Pilates. Others include Feldenkrais, Hellerwork, and the Alexander technique. Again, some of the skills may seem elementary, but your body may need to relearn them before you can progress because your brain may be stuck. Give it a try!

Feldenkrais. You may be asked to imagine different scenarios and then move your body in response. For example: lying face down, you may propel a steel ball down a groove that runs the full length of your body, using any muscles, but without changing position (Wildman, 1986).

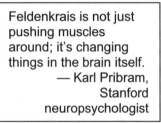

> Feldenkrais is not just pushing muscles around; it's changing things in the brain itself.
> — Karl Pribram, Stanford neuropsychologist

Hellerwork. This is a mind-body technique that combines deep-tissue muscle therapy, movement education, and massage.

Alexander technique. In this mind-body method to understand coordination, you observe your movement patterns and then, guided by an instructor, self-correct to eliminate unnecessary habits.

Pilates. In a class format, this mat exercise technique combines calisthenics and yoga to improve flexibility, strength, and balance, focusing on core strength. In private sessions, you'll use precise, slow movements on specialized equipment to develop muscle control.

Personal experience. While I've only heard recommendations about these other techniques, I joined a mat-Pilates class to see what was all the rage. Although it fully tested both my discipline and abdominals, I was bored because of the singular focus — I prefer variety. I also tried the Transformer, a special device which is used to stretch and strengthen the core of the body — the torso. Many people find the device very useful, but I decided that I could obtain the same benefits easier and faster without an instructor by weight training and stretching. Try — and see what works for you!

Other specialized programs like Brain Gym are available that focus on motion to improve brain functioning (Rogers & Brady, 1998).

What equipment is helpful?
Apparatus doesn't need to be expensive to work. While high-tech machines work and are fun, not using them doesn't mean that your improvement needs to stop at discharge. Daily practice with basic equipment will result in far greater gains than once-a-week training on high-tech devices. The key is practice-practice-practice.

Want to improve both balance and flexibility, while having fun? Roll either forward or backward on a large balance ball, lie on it both on your front and back, and play with it! You can also construct balance devices that work really well. See *Brain Injury Rewiring for Loved Ones,* Chapter 10, for directions.

Assistive devices support injured limbs and provide stability for walking, balancing, and lifting. Rather than feel embarrassed by your walker, cane, brace, or whatever you need, consider how much more embarrassed you'd feel if you fell! As your skills develop, use your device less.

Personal experience. In addition to the good-balance pose of my daily yoga "eagle," I still occasionally practice with a wooden balance board. Many years of practicing on it and walking on parking lot lines — despite funny looks — improved my equilibrium. Now I rarely fall from my bicycle and I can hold most yoga poses with just a bit of a waver. I'm also no longer asked to take "the drunk test" when stopped by the police! My favorite device is my balance ball, which serves as my desk chair, abdominal crunch device, and relaxer for hips and back — at any time of day! The disk-with-softball aids my balance so I can stand longer than a few seconds on my surfboard. Another day, another challenge!

Why is practice so important?
After our injuries, we may need to relearn movement skills the same way we originally learned them. And, we may need precise, successful practice —

> Showing up is 80 percent of life.
> — Woody Allen

thousands, even millions of times — to perfect the motor pattern (Kottke, 1980).

Sorry, survivors, but although new connections form during learning, we may need to practice for many months before these new connections develop and function (Rinehart, 1983). For the impatient among us, remember Dr. Kottke's practice rule: if it took three million steps to learn to walk, why expect that it would take any fewer to relearn to walk?

Fitness

After your balance and movement improve, you'll want to get fit. This involves strength, flexibility, and endurance — all three divided into frequency (how often), intensity (how hard), and duration (how long).

Strength

Let's look at what the word "strength" means: energy, force, vigor. Everything we do requires a certain amount of power, whether dressing or moving. Thus, to maximize our physical recovery and independence, we need to strength-train. Even drinking a beverage takes arm power — especially for those who are thirsty!

Are you worried about looking muscle-bound? No need. Those burly body builders found at every gym not only look in the mirror a lot, they also spend several hours every day lifting heavy weights. If you don't work out like them, you won't look like them.

When we strength-train, not only do our non-injured muscles gain vigor, but the affected ones may develop new *synapses* (nerve connections) from the stimulation that enable them to work — or work better. Stronger muscles also lead to greater cardiovascular gains. Another benefit of improved physical strength is increased self-esteem and confidence: "I can do this! Maybe I can do something else!"

Personal experience. *I know that new connections grow because I have experienced that since my injury in 1976. I remember one evening in the hospital psych ward when I cried out for a neurologist after my right arm collapsed as I attempted a push-up — I don't know why I was doing it; maybe I just had to see what I could do. Never before had my* *body failed me. I panicked. After a few cursory tests, I was told "you're not bad enough" for rehab.*

I knew my right side needed strengthening work, even if no one else did. So, as soon as I was released, I took myself to the local gym and started to lift weights. I could — and would — get stronger!

Deciding that the weak side needed to feel as if it belonged to my body, I allowed it to do extra. I didn't punish it for being weak — I rewarded it! For every additional repetition the right side did, I congratulated it — "Okay, good!" — And felt happy for small successes.

It took more than twenty years of work — but my right side nearly has caught up to my left side. I still sometimes let it do extra — and the results of constraint-induced movement therapy confirmed my results.

There is more in *Brain Injury Rewiring for Loved Ones,* Chapter 7.

How often should I do strength workouts? What frequency and duration?

Lifting every 48-96 hours gives your muscles time to repair. The two to four day range depends upon recovery from your previous workout, your energy level, and your age. To see what works best for

> Do one more than you think you can.
> — Raymond A. Dolen

your body, vary the amount of time between workouts. For example: a 60-minute workout on a tired day may feel as hard as a 90-minute workout on an energetic day.

If you're just starting — or resuming — lifting, 48 hours is probably enough time to recover after a 30-60 minute easy-to-moderate strength workout. If your workout is moderate and longer than 60 minutes, 72 hours is probably better. Age is another important consideration. Our muscles recover slower the older we get, so we need more time for muscle repair.

How do you know if it's enough recovery time? Listen to your body. If you don't want to work hard, go easy, go home, or go play!

How hard should I work? What is the right intensity?

Consider your goals: maintain minimal fitness, improve health, look good, compete with yourself or others, eat whatever you want — or a combination of these. Consult with the professionals on your health care team.

To strengthen our muscles, we need to challenge them. We also want to avoid injury. So, start with one set of 12-15 reps (repetitions). Depending on your goals, increase to 2-3 sets of 8-15 reps. Use a weight that you can lift with a moderate effort where the last two repetitions of any set are difficult but not painful. Work to fatigue. If completing 15 repetitions is easy, increase the weight the next time you lift. A typical rest period is 30-90 seconds between sets. A set may include 4-20 repetitions, with 12-15 the standard.

Why moderate, rather than easy? Because you gotta sweat, regardless of your goals. No effort means no benefit — a healthier version of "no pain, no gain." Sweating is a good indicator of effort.

What are various ways to work out?

If you seek variety and challenge, change your routine each time you lift — order, exercises, weights, equipment, length, or even the location — but always work your priority area first.

Options include super sets, pyramids, and various circuits. Because I don't like to waste time or be idle, my favorite is to super-set: perform two exercises in a row without rest, and then repeat. You can either work different or opposing muscle groups, varying the push-and-pull actions or upper- and lower-body parts. For example, a set of back exercises followed by a set of chest exercises or legs followed by chest.

Strength-training pyramids involve continuous lifting with increasing or decreasing amounts of weights and repetitions. For example: start with 15 repetitions with 12 pounds, then 12 repetitions with 10 pounds, then 10 repetitions with 8 pounds, then back up the ladder, decreasing repetitions and adding weight.

A circuit is a continuous session of non-stop exercises. It usually involves moving from one machine to the next, because machines are faster than free weights. A benefit of constantly moving is maintaining an elevated heart rate. Some gyms organize their machines in a circuit.

What's better — total-body workout or split routine?

This depends on your goals, motivation, time, and capacity. Doing a total-body strength workout of 12-15 exercises or machines every time you train, with two to four days in between, is usually easiest.

> My pleasure lies in seeing that I myself grow better day by day.
> — Epictetus

Some folks like to split their routine to focus on upper body one day and lower body the next. The advantage is a shorter and more concentrated workout. The disadvantage is the time commitment and possible burnout with this effort.

Strength training summary: the composition of a basic workout.
- Warm up till you're starting to perspire.
- Starting with your largest muscles, 10-20 exercises or machines.
- Warm down by stretching.

Monitor body and mind and change what isn't working — wear that scientist-hat! As you learn the basics, vary parts of the routine to suit your fitness goals and avoid boredom. If pressed for time, rather than skip a workout, shorten it. Perform one set for each large muscle group (chest, upper and lower back, abs, legs, arms). On those days when nothing seems to work, just play! Your body may need a break from a structured workout. Something is always better than nothing!

Flexibility

Do you want to enjoy physical activity — and sex — more? Stretch! To maximize muscle power, stretching is as important as strength training. It lengthens tight muscles, lubricates and cushions joints, increases range of motion, and reduces soreness from activity. Stretching can also help improve common stress-related disorders such as headache, insomnia, anxiety, and overeating (LeMay, 2003).

Whether we want to reach down and smell the roses or just get out of bed and dress, we need to bend and twist. Limber bodies move easier, perform better, and injure less frequently. Age and injury increase the value of flexibility because both decrease elasticity. Try this experiment:

skip stretching after a workout one day, then include stretching the next time. Which day-after feels better?

How do I stretch properly and how often?
Warm muscles like to stretch; cold ones don't — they may injure. So exercise to the point of sweating — at least five minutes, preferably ten. Then begin with your large muscles. Inhale before a stretch and exhale as you go into it and as you hold it. Then push a bit more air out, automatically inducing a deep inhalation. Stretch all muscle groups and focus on the muscle being stretched. Think top/bottom, left/right, up/down so nothing is skipped. Push to the edge of discomfort, but not to pain. Do not bounce! Bouncing is more likely to injure than help! The longer a stretch is held, the further you can push. Remember to breathe.

The traditional method involves holding a stretch for 10-60 seconds, relaxing, then repeating with different muscle groups. Another practice is called active isolated stretching (AIS) in which you first tighten the muscle opposite the one you want to stretch, hold for only two seconds, and then repeat 6-10 times. For example: to stretch the hamstrings, first tighten the quadriceps, which relaxes the hamstrings. The reasoning behind AIS is that the muscle will fight relaxation — the stretch reflex — if held for a longer period than 2 seconds.

Practicing yoga poses or using an exercise ball or belt or elastic tubing expands the variety of stretching possibilities. Be creative! Some days one technique will be more appealing and other days, another.

Stretching can also become part of a nightly relaxation/meditation time with music, at least three times a week. For optimum health, it's best to stretch daily!

Endurance

Are you short of breath from the effort of rising from your couch? How about after moving (walking, wheeling) a short distance at a leisurely pace? This is called cardiovascular deconditioning, lack of endurance, or simply being out of shape. Think "use it or lose it." Our heart and lungs respond to whatever level of work is required of them — no effort means no capacity. Our cardiovascular capacity determines our stamina.

How do we increase our endurance level? If we gradually increase the workload on our oxygen-delivery system, it responds by becoming stronger. The more regularly the stress is applied, the stronger and more durable we become — we can go longer at a faster pace without tiring.

What is aerobic exercise?

"Aerobic" mean "with air." So any repetitive activity that requires an extra supply of oxygen to move your muscles qualifies. Basically, any exercise that is done hard enough and long enough to challenge your heart and lungs to deliver oxygen to your muscles as you breathe is aerobic exercise. This includes house and yard work.

Lower-body exercises that use the large muscles of the legs, hips, and lower back all accomplish this goal. Examples include walking, running, swimming, stair-climbing, kicking, rowing, bicycling, and continuous weight training (circuit training).

Upper-body exercise that works the chest, back, and arms provides similar benefits. Examples include various indoor and outdoor wheelchair options, water sports, circuit training, and indoor equipment such as stationary arm bikes.

What is anaerobic exercise?

When your muscles demand more oxygen than your heart and lungs can deliver, you are anaerobic or "without air." Gasping for breath and feeling a burning sensation in your muscles (from lactic acid buildup) signal that you are at your anaerobic threshold.

Naturally, the lower your fitness level, the sooner you reach this level. As your body adapts to higher exercise workloads, it becomes more efficient at taking in oxygen — allowing you to breathe and work at the same time! This adaptation period is called training. People train for all sorts of things such as triathlons and our bodies become stronger in response to greater demands on them.

How do I know how hard I'm working? What the intensity of my work is?

Several methods gauge your exertion level: the talk test, perceived exertion, and your heart rate.

> Start by doing what's necessary, then what's possible and suddenly you are doing the impossible.
> — St. Francis of Assisi

The talk test is the simplest method. If you can carry on a conversation during exercise — even a few words aloud to yourself — you're working at a light-to-moderate level.

Rating perceived exertion requires you to numerically evaluate how hard you feel you're working, on a scale from 1 to 10. For example, a rating of 1 may correspond to sitting or lying, a 3 might be a leisurely stroll, a 5 walking or rolling at a moderate pace, 7 the start of the "hard" level such as running, wheeling, or cycling over rolling hills. An all-out effort qualifies as a 10 — maybe a 20-second burst in a race or the last few yards of an uphill sprint. Using this gauge, an aerobic effort probably falls between levels 4 and 8. To measure perceived exertion, evaluate your breathing or sweating rate or how tired your muscles feel — whatever works for you to determine effort.

As fitness increases, any effort appears easier, so after a few weeks what started out feeling like an 8 may feel like a 4. Raise your intensity level to continue to strengthen your oxygen transport system.

To measure heart rate we count the number of times the heart beats per minute. Use a heart-rate monitor or do it manually: during or after exercise, stand by a clock or look at a watch. Place your index and middle fingers gently either against your carotid artery on your neck (in the groove under your jaw) or the inner side of your wrist by the tendons. Don't use your thumb because it has its own pulse. When the second hand reaches a starting number you'll remember such as 12 or 6, watch for at least 15 seconds. Either count the beats for 15 seconds and multiply by 4 or count for 30 seconds and multiply by 2 for beats per minute. Count for a full minute on a digital watch or buy a heart rate monitor and check it every five to ten minutes.

Counting for less than 15 seconds isn't accurate because your heart rate decreases rapidly as soon as you stop exercising, so one beat makes a big difference. The fitter you are, the faster your heart rate drops. Within the first minute, the heart rate of someone in good shape will drop at least 40 beats. *Here's another goal!*

Why do I want to know how hard I'm working?

The purpose of listening to our body's signals is to measure our workout intensity so we obtain the results we want. Part of this whole rewiring process is to maximize our potential in the shortest time possible, right?

> The only thing that ever sat its way to success was a hen.
> — Sarah Brown

For example, if your pulse beats 25 times in fifteen seconds, that's 100 beats per minute, which is probably at the low end of your exercise range, may feel like a 3 on the perceived exertion scale, and enables you to sing a rock song at full volume. In other words, the exercise is not hard enough to obtain benefits for most of us.

How do I determine my target heart rate?

Several methods that vary in difficulty and accuracy can predict a range of numbers that suggest a zone in which to work for maximum cardiovascular benefits.

The age-based maximum heart rate is well known, easiest, and the most inaccurate method to estimate target heart rate. To calculate, first subtract your age from 220 for males or 226 for females. Multiply the result by 65% for the low end of your range and by 85% for the high end. Or use whatever percentages you and your doctors choose.

For example: take a 20-year old man: 220 minus 20 is 200. Sixty-five percent of 200 is 0.65 X 200 = 130 and eighty-five percent of 200 is 0.85 X 200 = 170. Using this method, our guy needs to work out at between 130 and 170 beats per minute. If he works out at a lower level than this, the benefits are few; if higher, he'll probably need to take a break for air. Working out at too high an intensity can actually decrease fitness. Cells are damaged by overuse and *free radicals* can overwhelm the *antioxidants* when you overexert.

The **Karvonen formula** is another age-based method. While a bit more complicated, this method is more accurate because an individual's resting heart rate is also taken into consideration along with age.

Let's say our 20-year old guy has a resting heart rate (upon awakening) of 70 beats per minute. We start the same way, subtracting his age from 220 (220 minus 20 = 200), then subtract his resting heart rate from that result (200 minus 70 = 130). Then, 65% of 130 is 0.65 X 130 = 0.85 (rounded). Multiply this number by 100, which gives 85. Finally, to determine the low end of his range, add his resting heart rate to this number: 85 + 70 = 155. Similarly, to determine the high end of his range, find 85% of 130 (0.85 X 130 = 111), add his resting heart rate to the result (111 + 70 = 181). Thus, 181 is the high end of his range. If our 20-year-old targets this range for his workout — between 155 and 181 beats per minute — he'll work out at an appropriate level, thus attaining more cardiovascular fitness.

Other methods rely on the expertise of professionals and their equipment. For example, a trainer may ask you to strap on a heart-rate monitor and then jump on an arm or leg bike, Stairmaster, or treadmill and gradually increase your intensity every three to four minutes for about 15 minutes. Trained medical personnel may also test your absolute maximum, but it doesn't feel good! You may want to consult with your health professionals and set a goal together.

What's the lesson here?
Listen to your own body and use the formulas as guides. Only you know how hard you can go. What happens if you go too hard? Your fitness level decreases. When you are exhausted, you set yourself up for significant injuries that really eat into your training time. The intensity levels are set for a reason — following them is the best way to achieve maximum fitness.

Why measure heart rate before arising in the morning?
Resting heart rate is more than a gauge of fitness — it also indicates the status of your body's repair process. Let's say, for example, that today your heart beats ten or more beats faster than yesterday. This is a signal that your body has not recovered from whatever occurred yesterday —

whether it was work, play, or other stress. *Stress can be positive or negative!*

So, is a higher heart rate an excuse to sleep in and avoid exercise? Nope. It is simply a warning — like a yellow light — that if you push hard today and are exposed to anyone's sickness, you're at increased risk for illness or injury. A healthy response is to do moderate activity, pay attention to your body's signals, and — if possible — stay away from the coughers and sneezers. After some listen-to-your-body experiences, you'll tune in to the signals and know how to stay healthy.

A slow pulse (heart rate) is good. Resting heart rate in some elite athletes may be as slow as 35-45 beats per minute (BPM). Most people are in the 70-80 BPM range. Genetics plays a role in this, so don't feel like a failure if you work out hard and your resting pulse remains in the 50s.

Personal experience. After over thirty years of body signals, I'm finally listening better. I used to ignore the signals, go ahead with my intended gut-busting workouts anyway, and get so sick I couldn't work out for a week. After a few hundred repetitions of this — and my best friend's reminders — I now usually slow down and heed this message: "Either do less today or none for the next week. What do you want?" I still test myself now and again because I am a survivor and an athlete.

How can I measure progress?
Performing a timed test of any exercise is a good way. First, warm up for 5-10 minutes. Then walk, wheel, run, or skate for a measured distance. If you prefer a bicycle or a chair, ride for five miles. If swimming is your favorite, time yourself for 500 yards/meters. To track fitness improvements, test yourself monthly and record the time. Naturally, as fitness and speed increase, time decreases. It's you against the clock!

What frequency and duration do I need to improve my endurance?
Aim for a daily 30-90 minutes of moderate exercise. If long (30 minutes or more) sessions are too difficult at the beginning, do 10-15 minute sessions. Any sustained activity — even 10 minutes at a time — will increase your fitness.

Improving your health requires at least thirty minutes of activity five days a week. Thirty minutes, three days a week, provides minimum maintenance, but improvement requires more. *Don't we want to get better?*

> It is a happy talent to know how to play.
> — Ralph Waldo Emerson

Exercise Equipment Ideas

Indoor cardiovascular conditioning and strength. Use leg and arm bicycles, portable leg exercisers, treadmills, stair-steppers, elliptical trainers, rowing machines, and cross-country ski machines. Jump rope! Even using cleaning devices like brooms, vacuums, and mops works — if done long enough.

Outdoor cardiovascular. Try bicycles, racing chairs, and various water toys such as kayaks, body boards, canoes. Walk with light hand-weights. Garden, work with tools like a rake, shovel, or broom.

Indoor strength training, flexibility, and balance. Use a variety of free weights, machines, and devices that include mats, the floor, walls, balls, stairs, benches, balance boards or discs, hand weights, stretch cords, pulleys, pull-up bars, towels, broomsticks, or chairs — whatever works!

Where do I find reasonably priced equipment?

Ask your local sporting goods stores about used equipment. Look in the want ads and the phone book. Go to thrift shops and yard sales.

Personal experience. Needing a quick morning pick-up, I found a brand-name stair stepper for $8.99 at a local thrift shop! It's a great way to raise my metabolic rate in throughout the day 10-15 minute sessions— or longer, if weather interferes with my usual outdoor activities.

Workout Attire

Choosing clothes and shoes for workouts isn't a girl thing — really! It can make the difference between enjoying wh it you're doing — or not. Workout clothes made from microfiber fabric that wicks perspiration are best because they're lightweight and they breathe. Cotton becomes heavy when soaked and stays wet, which can lead to a chill. Some clothes are specially designed for certain activities. For example, tight-fitting bicycle shorts compress and stabilize leg muscles so they function better when asked to work hard.

Shoes also need to be chosen for the activity. For example, running shoes are not good for weight training because they don't provide lateral stability. Likewise, shoes for weight training are not good for running, although cross trainers work OK for most sports. Walking and running shoes differ in the placement of their cushioning. Special bicycle shoes with a firm platform transfer your power to the pedal, rather than wasting it by flexing as tennis shoes do. If you don't want to waste money, watch for sales and buy at discount houses and thrift stores.

Facilities and Resources

To decide where to work out, analyze your needs and resources so you'll follow through and meet your goals. Ask yourself: "Will I really go to a gym?" and "Will I exercise at home in front of the TV when I'd rather sit on the couch and eat?" Then consider interest, cost-effectiveness, convenience, and social and health benefits.

Interest

Home. To exercise at home sounds great, but is it, really? So, try before you buy. Visit a local fitness store and use different machines with the clothes you'll wear when you work out. Wear your headphones. Then ask yourself, "Do I like it and will I use it every day for 30 minutes or longer?" With a multi-use machine, "Do I want to change all that apparatus for different muscle groups every time I work out?"

Gym. To find one you'll use regularly, trust your instincts. Ask:
- How do I feel when I'm here?
- Is the facility and equipment in good shape?
- Do I want classes or just equipment?
- Do the classes appeal to me?
- Is the staff friendly?
- Do I feel comfortable with the people who work out here?
- Is the lighting adequate?

- Is it spacious?
- If you use a chair, are the machines accessible?
- Is the gym crowded at the times when I'll use it?

An advantage survivors usually have is that we can go during afternoon hours that are less busy — and often at a reduced rate.

Facilities typically offer various classes at different levels, lots of exercise apparatus in several rooms, and professional assistance. Tennis/racquetball and basketball courts, swimming pools, Jacuzzi/steam/sauna rooms, and childcare are often available as well. Some local health clubs may even provide television and Internet hookups or compact-disc changers on some cardio equipment.

Convenience

Home. Ask:
- What do I need for a complete workout?
- Is my equipment located so I can use it easily?
- Where does it go when not in use?

Gym. Ask:
- Is it close enough to me so that I'll go?
- How's the traffic and parking?
- How will I get there?

Cost

Home. To exercise at home may sound more economical, but is it really? Investing in exercise equipment, whether new or used, may not be the best use of resources. Will it be used? Are you motivated to do it with no one around for company? A complete home-exercise program requires free weights and/or a multi-station weight machine, as well as cardiovascular equipment such as an Exercycle. Just one piece of quality equipment can cost four times as much as a yearly membership to a local health club or gym. And that piece of exercise equipment can become very boring.

As far as television infomercials and other advertised exercise products go, don't buy sight unseen! As appealing as those ads seem, the equipment usually fails to live up to promises, costs more than it's worth, is a pain to return, gathers dust, and wastes money.

Health club. What is included in the cost of a gym membership? Dues can range from $99 per year for a bare-bones club to many times that amount for a full-service club with many classes. One option is to choose a basic membership plan and pay for special classes separately. Ask about scholarships — YMCAs often offer these — and trial memberships. Can the monthly fee be suspended for injury and/or sickness?

When comparing exercise costs, determine which classes you're likely to take. Then figure the costs of the same classes from outside sources. For example: if you're a swimmer, what's the fee to swim at a pool? Or, what is the cost of yoga, karate, or other classes at another facility? Although initial costs appear higher, a full-service club is usually far cheaper. We're also more likely to go if it's already paid for!

Personal experience. I love health clubs! I'm greeted the moment I arrive, enjoy every minute, and only feel sad when I need to leave.

Social and Health Benefits

With social interaction so vital for our health, going to a gym offers distinct advantages over working out at home. There's a special feeling of camaraderie among exercisers — we respect others who also sweat and exert. We all understand what it takes to do what we do. We're disciplined and committed to self-improvement. Gyms are also great places to meet members of the opposite sex with similar interests, whether we participate in classes or work out at a regular time.

And, on those days when it's an effort just to get there, some wonderful thing will happen or someone will compliment us. At the very least, we burn calories and are productive!

Exercise Questions and Answers

Burning calories and losing fat.
Exercising our muscles improves how we look like nothing else can! Here's a bonus — we don't burn calories only when we exercise!

Increased calorie burning occurs all day long when we increase our muscle mass. Why? Active tissue like muscle fiber demands more energy than inactive tissue like fat. More energy means burning more calories. Our calorie-burning furnaces burn hotter for hours after we finish our exercise. The number of hours depends on the intensity — how hard we exercise, and the duration — how long we exercise. Consider the lean physiques of active children and teens.

What about pace? Is it better to work slow and long?
The concept of a preferred fat-burning zone is controversial. Here's why: while exercise at a lower level of intensity burns a greater percentage of stored fat than recently consumed carbohydrates, more

> The distance doesn't matter; only the first step is difficult.
> — Mme. du Deffand

total calories — and thus more fat — is burned at higher levels of intensity.

Consider: if someone pedaled an Exercycle at a leisurely pace that burned 100 calories in 30 minutes, about 80%, or 80 calories, might be fat calories. If our slowpoke picked up the pace to burn 300 calories, then 30%, about 90 fat-calories, are zapped. While a smaller percentage, three times as many total calories and 10 additional fat calories are burned.

So, is a fast pace the best way to go? No — not if you can only sustain it for a few minutes. The goal is to just do it — even if slow is the only way you can go! More calories and more fat are burned at a slow pace than at no pace! Eventually you'll be able to increase the intensity. On those days when a hard pace is too hard, reduce the effort. It's better to walk leisurely on your treadmill than to hang clothes on it. Better slow than no!

What is the right pace to improve my health?
It depends on your goals. To minimally strengthen your cardiovascular system takes just a little effort. For example: if you want to be able to walk or wheel to the corner without needing a breather, then exercising at a low level of intensity three days a week for thirty minutes a day is all you need.

If, however, you want to be able to walk/wheel across the parking lot to your car and then carry several loads of groceries from the car without resting, you'll need to do more — perhaps thirty minutes five days a week at a moderate level of intensity. If you'd like a trim-looking body, it'll take still more, such as 60 minutes a day of moderate-to-hard varied activity that includes strength training. And, if racing is on your mind,

> I run because I am an animal and a child, an artist and a saint. So, too, are you. Find your own play, your own self-renewing compulsion, and you will become the person you are meant to be.
> — George Sheehan, MD

we're talking about various modes of exercise at a moderate-to-hard level for about 15 hours a week, depending on your current levels.

Activity Suggestions

Participate to the extent of your ability and remember: do anything and practice-practice-practice!

Learning tips:
- Because of the memory impairment and auditory processing problems that we typically experience, you'll probably find that any activity is easier and more fun with some kind of direction, like audio or video tapes, if no personal instruction is available.
- Partnering with someone also doubles the fun and decreases the perception of work!
- To move the memory of a new physical skill to a permanent storage site in the brain requires at least six hours, even for those without injury. When a new skill was attempted in less than six hours, the first one may be erased (Liu, 1997).

Indoor

For individual or group activities, on the floor, in chairs, or in the pool, consider:
- Land or water aerobics.
- Swimming classes or programs.

- Low- or high-impact cardiovascular floor movements.
- Spinning on a stationary bicycle or on a trainer with a road bike.
- Cardio machines, such as rower, elliptical, stair-stepper, treadmill.
- Weight training
- Walking programs — offered by many shopping malls.
- Dancing: swing, salsa, ballroom, ballet, jazz, tap, etc.
- Martial arts like karate, kung fu, or kickboxing.
- Jumping rope.
- Yoga, tai chi, Qigong, stretches.
- Balancing activities using large balls, etc.

Personal experience. After failing at my pre-injury favorites, I was willing to try something else — anything else! Karate was one of my first successful athletic endeavors after my injury, probably because precise balance is unnecessary and it involves only a few slow moves at the beginning. I later enjoyed tai chi, especially to help me focus for a race.

To improve eye-hand coordination:
- Juggle anything. Start with something soft and easy like scarves. With mastery, move to balls, starting with two.
- Play paddleball with yourself! To start, use paddles with attached balls. They're fun and productive — no hunting for an errant ball! With mastery, play table tennis (ping-pong). Begin by tilting the table to use as a backboard, then add a live partner.

> Good for the body is the work of the body, and good for the soul is the work of the soul, and good for either is the work of the other.
> — Henry David Thoreau

Outdoor

Land sports:
- Bicycling, wheeling, skating — wear guards and helmet.
- Gardening and other yard work — both productive and fun!
- Running or walking Nature journeys — act like a tourist in your area.

- Ball/missile sports: tennis, Frisbee, croquet. Play catch!
- Kite flying — energetic or relaxed.

Water sports:
- Swimming: pool and open water. Safeguards include swimming where there are lifeguards, with buddies, in known conditions, wearing bright yellow caps, and coming in when cold or tired.
- Body boarding (boogie boarding), board and kayak surfing.
- Kayaking, canoeing, rowing — wear a helmet in surf!

> Climb the mountains and get their good tidings. Nature's peace will flow into you as sunshine flows into trees. The winds will blow their freshness into you, and the storms their energy, while cares will drop off like falling leaves.
> — John Muir

Adapted Activities

Loss of full mobility doesn't need to mean loss of active fun! Ask your physical therapist to show you ways to adapt equipment. Various assistive straps, etc. are available for weight training, for example. While participation in activities is more complicated for users of supportive devices, fun is still on the agenda. Be creative! Here are some ideas:
- Any exercise equipment or machine, arm cycles.
- Balancing and strengthening activities that use a ball.
- Bicycling with adapted equipment or on a tandem or recumbent bike.
- Outdoor water sports like sit-on-top water skis, kayaks, outrigger canoes.
- Indoor water sports and aquatic activities.
- Snow sports with modified skis and sleds.
- Wheelchair sports like basketball, quad rugby, tennis, volleyball.
- Chair dancing.
- Gardening with adaptive techniques and equipment.

Accessible Gardening

Use a wheelchair? Not a problem! Just adapt the bed and pathway design and use adaptive tools — presto, you're out there gardening! Your interest and aptitude for gardening may even lead to a new career!

Manual skills such as strength, coordination, mobility, flexibility, and dexterity are required to garden. See how simply and easily physical rehabilitation can happen? If you have mobility and limb impairments, learn how to use adaptive equipment and work in raised garden settings. See *Brain Injury Rewiring for Loved Ones,* Chapter 10, for more.

Competitive Sports

Racers in lightweight chairs continually set new records at various distances, whether using arm cycles in bicycle races or racing chairs on running courses. Triathlons also accommodate wheelchair users and offer categories for various disabilities. The Paralympic Games also offer many ways to compete. The next Paralympics is 2012 in London, so get ready!

If you want the action of extreme sports, you're in luck! The Extremity Games began in 2006, just for you! Similar to the X-Games, this competition is for athletes with amputations and limb differences. Awards include medals as well as prizes and money! For newcomers, instructional clinics are also held in each of the sports, which include: BMX, kayaking, motocross, mountain biking, rock climbing, skateboarding, surfing, and wakeboarding. What fun! See the *Brain Injury Rewiring for Loved Ones* Resources for website information.

> It's no longer a focus on the disability. It's a focus on the possibility.
> — Dr. Joanne Westphal

If you want a free machine of any type, apply to the Challenged Athletes Foundation (CAF). It sponsors events to raise money for disabled athletes and only requires a compelling application from you! *A few years ago I earned a nice $1000 grant toward a custom-designed racing bicycle.*

Personal experience. *Neither snow nor hail — nor flat tires — keeps me from that finish line! I'll always remember a triathlon on Camp*

Pendleton, the local Marine base. As I descended the last hill, feeling fast, I looked down at my computer, happily noting my speed of 39 mph. Then I heard a psst-like air explosion. Yep — flat tire.

> There are two ways you can go. You can continue life and keep going or you can go home and vegetate.
> — Don Hyslop
> (wheelchair racer)

The good news was I knew how far I was from the finish line because my computer registered distance — only 3.5 miles! I can push my bike that far! Anyone who's worn or seen bicycle shoes knows that I needed to remove them to make progress, so I walked/ran in my new socks.

Everyone who passed encouraged me, but since the women started last, now I really was last! The Marines who rode in the sweep vehicle asked me many times. "Hey, lady, are you sure you don't want a ride?" Because our ages are marked on our legs, they knew my age (50) and probably considered that someone as old as their mothers might want some help. Perhaps they wanted to finish their jobs. Whatever, I graciously declined their offers of a ride and they cheered my every step.

As I finally reached the transition area, I saw a friend of mine who told me her kids were on their bikes looking for me on the running course. Now I had another goal! They found me and rode along with me as I ran the three miles, happily in shoes this time. We set the goal of passing the only two people still on the course. As I ran faster, they ran faster. Alas, the distance was too short for me to catch them! They crossed the finish line about 15 yards ahead of me!

Yes, I finished last — but I finished. And I won a case of beer — we called it the "inspirational award." More than that, I regained my pride. I was not a quitter. Brain injury or not, nothing can stop me now. Sometimes "it is darkest before the dawn."

The post-injury challenge. As we all know, our injuries affect our abilities in sports, just like in everything else. And, regardless of our previous level, we're simply not as good. We can be better than we are, but comparing ourselves to what we were probably creates stress. Do we still want to pursue old favorites?

Maybe we need a change, continuing to participate, but playing with different goals — fun?! — and maybe even trying new sports!

Personal experience. I used to love to play singles tennis, but when I tried to play post-injury, I failed miserably. What to do? I still wanted to play, so I bought a new large-face racquet, took lessons, practiced with a ball machine, and tried doubles. It didn't help. I still played poorly — and ended up stressed, rather than relaxed. So I gave tennis a rest for about twenty years and built my strength and endurance through other sports. Now I pursue tennis only during the off-season from triathlon and mostly with people who just want to hit. When I play for points, if it becomes stressful, I stop. Enjoyment is now the name of the game.

While I miss my former successes, I find new ones to enjoy. Now, when I participate in races, I don't really compete against others. I just pit myself against the clock or the ocean or road or mountain — or nothing! — And I'm much happier. Now I just do it! — for play!

Relaxation Activities

Total health depends on wellness of body, mind, and spirit. We know that our emotions affect our physical health and that chronic stress impairs this system. Stress hormones can even kill memory-associated brain cells! Depression may lead to bodily changes that make us susceptible to disease because depleted immunity increases our chances of illness (Moyers, 1993).

Okay, we know all this. We also know that we need to relax. When our *chi* flows freely, we're balanced. Relaxation reduces stress and enhances immune functioning. Our health depends on our relaxing. But how?

Various cultures through the ages relaxed in vastly different ways. Just as there are many paths up the spiritual and therapeutic mountains, so are there many paths up the relaxation mountain. We'll look at the most widely practiced, yoga, which comes from the Indian tradition, and follow with its cousin from the Chinese tradition, Qigong. By focusing on breath and slow movements, anyone — regardless of physical abilities — can benefit from these practices.

Yoga

We've probably all seen pictures of an old guy with a peaceful expression sitting in what looks like a very painful position. How can this be? He's doing Hatha yoga, in which body-mind-spirit union is primarily achieved through a series of postures and breathing exercises. Depending on the setting, sacred sounds are also used.

How can yoga heal and relax me?

Postures massage glands, organs, and the endocrine system, which increases circulation and aids in eliminating toxins from the body. Postures also increase flexibility of muscles, tendons, and ligaments, relieving back pain. Relaxation occurs because the stretching, breathing, and guided relaxation of yoga release bodily tension and calm the nervous system and emotions. You also sleep and remember better!

What are the styles of Hatha yoga?

Beginners should consider these styles:

- Viniyoga was developed for those with injuries. Postures are modified to meet individual needs. This approach emphasizes the breath and is less technical than Iyengar and gentler than Ashtanga.
- Iyengar focuses strongly on alignment using props and emphasizes the therapeutic properties of poses.
- Kripalu is a gentle, therapeutic, and spiritually focused yoga with clear alignment that uses a three-stage approach and meditation within the yoga poses.

Other yoga styles — not recommended for beginners — include:

- Ashtanga/power, an athletic and fast-paced style, using a rigid sequence of poses.
- Bikram/hot, also athletic and physically focused, is practiced in a room heated to over 100 degrees! Bikram uses a rigid series of poses and instructors typically encourage students to push past limits (www.yogabasics.com, 2005).

Personal experience. When I lived in Mission Beach (a part of San Diego, California) in the 1980s, everybody did yoga, so I joined in, too! I found peace and relaxation and learned stretches that aided my triathlon

competition. Whether videos, classes, or practicing by myself, I continue
to use yoga daily to heal and relax.

Qigong and Tai Chi

Want to relax and get healthier without a lot of sweat and effort? Try the
moving meditations of qigong (pronounced "chee gong") or tai chi.
Doing "the big dance" improves strength, balance, flexibility, and
endurance, reduces the risk of falls and lowers blood pressure. If you're
easily distracted, participation can improve focus, discipline, memory,
and self-esteem, as well as decrease stress.

Doing qigong or tai chi for just thirty minutes four days a week
provides the same benefits as other moderate-intensity exercise such as
low-impact aerobics and brisk walking. And, by strengthening the joint
musculature and increasing range of motion and flexibility, these
activities may also help those who struggle with arthritis (Roach, 1997;
Moline, 1998).

In class, participants practice a sequence of very slow, ballet-like
movements, appearing almost in a trance as they concentrate on their
breathing. Qigong flows through about 15 moves, each with a colorful
name like Pushing the Wave, in a meditation that takes about 15 to 20
minutes. It is sometimes called "internal yoga" for its combination of
self-massage, snail-paced movement, breathing exercises, and
meditation. Those who practice regularly claim that it boosts their
vitality, improves their health, and helps them relax because the energy
change affects everything. Tai chi goes through a longer form with
similar goals. These Chinese practices that harmonizes *qi* (*chi*) can be
learned from a coach, book, or video (Evans, 1997).

My Progress to Date

I believe the just-do-it and practice-practice-practice adages. And I did it!
Currently, my goal is to make Team USA in triathlon to compete in the
world championship race held yearly. Because it's age-grouped in five-
year increments, there's always hope! All I need to do is compensate for
paralyzed and weak shoulder muscles. Someday, I may also compete in

an Ironman — preferably the Hawaii Ironman Triathlon. If not, my journey will show many smaller victories of mind and body.

Despite frequent injuries from overuse and crashing, I continue my quest, athletic and otherwise, to be all I can be. Although my injury-proneness is likely brain-injury-related — same drive, different ability, I have no visible disability. Thus, I compete with able-bodied athletes in all my races. I cycle on roads, trails, and in velodromes. I run, swim, board- and kayak-surf, and compete in triathlons.

For 20 years post-injury only occasionally was I seen anywhere near the victory podium — most times my pace was painfully slow at the end. But I always finished, so I kept training and

> Practice is the best of all instructors.
> — Publilius Syrus

occasionally raced when I wasn't injured. That's all God wanted for me, anyway — never to quit on my way to the Ultimate Accounting. Now, more than 30 years post-injury, I'm winning some races because so few of my age are still doing it! Persevere!

Self-Care

While exercise invigorates us, it also awakens some sleeping body parts. This section explains what you can do to care for those newly revived muscles. Listen to your body say, "Hello brain. Here I am. Tend to me!"

Acute Injuries

Assessment. Is the pain or soreness in the muscle or in a bone or joint? If it's severe pain from a bone, a joint, or your head, seek medical attention. Here's a clue: bone injuries usually swell up immediately. If it's a minor joint sprain, muscle strain, or soreness, treat it yourself first and monitor it.

Treatment. As soon as possible, to relieve pain and swelling of overstretched tissues and promote healing and flexibility, use RICE: Rest, Ice, Compression, and Elevation.

Rest means to stop using it to give it a chance to heal. Continuing to use the injured or sore area makes it worse.

Ice reduces pain and decreases swelling. Immediately apply an ice pack for 10-20 minutes or massage with ice — paper cups containing ice work well. Repeat every 2-3 hours for 48 hours. Do not apply an ice pack directly to skin — place a light cloth over it. While heat may feel better at first, it actually increases inflammation and swelling — so don't use heat!

Compression means to wrap the injured area with an elastic bandage such as an Ace wrap to apply pressure to reduce swelling. Don't wrap so tightly that it tingles, hurts, or is numb. Wear for at least 48 hours.

Elevation means to raise the injured body part above your heart, when possible, to help reduce swelling. Do this when applying ice or any time you sit or lie down. Elevation helps to drain any accumulated fluid from the injured area.

Chronic Injuries

Different from a recent injury, a chronic injury is one that either keeps returning or never leaves! In addition to seeking help from professionals, you may want to self-massage and use pressure-point therapy. To keep playing and prevent soreness after activity, wrap with an ice pack. A variety of ice packs to form-fit different body parts are available.

Self-Massage

Muscles perform better when they're relaxed. The job of self-care is to relax these tight muscles. Utilizing both pressure-point techniques and various strokes, self-massage can relax specific tight muscles, alleviate general soreness, and energize the whole body. Here are various feel-good techniques:

Shoulders: Using the opposite hand, cross it in front of your chest and apply pressure in circular motions as deeply as you can tolerate — the deeper the better. Repeat on your other side.

Chest: Using your thumbs, apply pressure with a circular motion to sensitive areas.

Legs: From a seated position, first apply thumb pressure with circular strokes to sore areas. Then, using your hand, stroke toward the heart with as much pressure as desired. Do on each leg.

Arms: From a seated position, with arms raised, stroke downward toward your heart, starting at your hand. Then, cross muscle fibers with a twisting motion. Repeat on your other arm.

Feet: Using both thumbs, apply circular pressure to sensitive areas, then stroke back and forth with knuckles. Stretch each toe.

Hands: Using thumb, apply circular pressure to sensitive areas, then stroke toward your heart with your knuckles. Pinch the webbed area between your thumb and forefinger. Stretch each finger.

Face: Using fingers, first stroke across both eyebrows. Then apply pressure to both temples with circular strokes. Repeat on both sides of your nose, mouth, and around each eye socket. Then work your fingers around each ear, both inside and outside. Pinch both ear lobes at several points.

Pressure-Point Therapy

Using the pad of your middle finger or your thumb, apply pressure wherever soreness is felt. Avoid any area of scar tissue, infection, or bruising. If in doubt, ask a professional to help you.

- **Time:** hold for 1-5 minutes per point or until relief is felt.
- **Pressure:** as much as tolerated.
- **Method:** start with small, circular movements. Progress to deep, constant pressure.

Summary

I hope and pray that you, too, will utter the "I will" and "I can" words. Maybe not sooner, but definitely not later. Maybe weakly at first, then tentatively — and later, perhaps even vigorously!

Or not. Maybe you won't say them at all — you'll just do it! That's fine, because my mission will be accomplished if you act! Remember: behavior change precedes attitude change. Here's what I

> You're never a loser until you quit trying.
> — Mike Ditka

propose: just do it! And practice-practice-practice! Following these two refrains won't bring back the way you were, but you'll be the best you can be. And, even when you stumble — and you will — give it a go before you say no!

Remember:
- Just do it!
- Find out what activities you like — and do one or two daily.
- Schedule activities on your calendar.
- Do relaxation activities like yoga, Qigong, or tai chi.
- Use RICE (Rest, Ice, Compression, Elevate), pressure-point, and self-massage techniques.

11

Social Rewiring:
Healing Our Spirits with
People Connections

I was naturally socially at ease until the
accident; after that I didn't know what to do or
what was wrong. It was just obvious that
something was very wrong — and I was that
something.
— Carolyn E. Dolen, 1976

Does my despair sound familiar? Most aware survivors echo a similar
lament. We were better before the injury, nothing is right anymore, and
we are the problem. Few people disagree with us.

Although views of the dilemma — and how to fix it — often differ,
others with whom we interact — from the checker at the local grocery
store to family members and friends — see a problem, too. Maybe the
fault isn't with what we are, but rather with what we do.

Whatever it is that we do, it produces a hail of sparks that reach
everywhere we go. Working with our rewiring team, we can locate the
problem areas and reinforce, reroute, and rebuild connections. Behavior
can change, so I revised my 1976 plea of *"Fix my brain and I won't be
crazy!"* to a new plan of *"Let us seek an error to correct rather than a*

fault to criticize." This chapter explores the why, what, and how of social rewiring, with behaviors to fix and strategies for repair. We discuss:

- The importance of social ties.
- Social challenges.
- SAFER — Stop, Assess, Fix, Evaluate, Retry.
- Relationship changes.
- Dating.
- Sex.
- Relearning social skills: strategies and activities.

Introduction

"Okay, world, here I come! I've waited long enough. It's now or never. — But wait! I don't feel quite ready. Why? Why don't I feel okay yet? I've worked so hard. So, why am I not fixed?

"I've been assessed, analyzed, and linked to every machine in the hospital and rehab center! I've been subjected to X-rays, MRIs, EKGs, CT scans, and ICPs. I've even been PETed. I've been IVed and cathed, stapled and stitched, pricked and probed, trached and vented. I've swallowed medications of every size, shape, and color. I'm in tumult. Every part of me feels twisted and tweaked, needled and noodled.

"I've tried every therapy invented. I've seen neurologists for my neurons, psychiatrists for my psyche, and cognitive specialists for my comprehension. Physical therapists train my body; speech therapists teach my brain. Music and massage minister to my soul and psychologists mend my mind. Occupational therapists adjust my limbs and recreational therapists teach me to play.

"I'm equipped with hearing aids to block noise, lenses to diffuse light, and magnets to free my bioelectricity. My feet are corrected with orthotics and my legs are braced with the latest Velcro and plastic. I'm rewired, rehabilitated, and ready to venture forth into the world, right?"

Well, maybe — not!

"But why not? I bathe, toilet, shave, dress, and feed myself. I brush my teeth and comb my hair. I wear deodorant and clean clothes. I don't usually spit, curse, or make loud noises. Look where I've been! Look how far I've come! Why aren't I ready? After all I've done…"

Well, folks, it's about that rewiring. God didn't construct us the second time around. Now we're imperfect. With the damage to our main transformer, wires may be frayed, hidden, shorted, or disconnected. Others may be lost. And, despite everyone's best efforts, some wires remain crossed. A few need more insulation, while others need less. Heaven forbid — but we may even be overwired! Many of us look ready to socialize, but we're not. Some of us may never be totally ready, and most of us are ready only some of the time. But, if we continue to work on our social skills, they will improve. If not, they won't.

"Okay, then they won't. I'll just be alone. It's too much trouble to be around people. And besides, no one understands. Nobody needs me and I don't need anybody else! Socializing is too hard! Other people take energy that I can't spare — I have enough troubles of my own to deal with. I'll be fine — I can heal myself. Please, just leave me alone!"

Importance of Social Ties

Being Alone — What Happens?

If we choose to withdraw and be alone, will we really be fine? The alone time that we want can lead to loneliness that we don't want, which can spiral to despair — and even death. To capture the same joy that humans can provide, we try food, drink, drugs, and/or tobacco. Depression does that! We seek first one thing and then another to quench our hunger for love.

To test the idea that isolation accelerates aging and death, nearly 5000 people were followed for nine years. The mortality rate for those without social ties was double that for those with the strongest social links, leading to the conclusion that loneliness kills more people than any other disease (Sobel & Ornstein, 1998).

Social Interactions Equal Health

How does loneliness kill? Isolation leads to early death, both from disease processes and from suicide (Teasdale and Engberg, 2001). Decades of research conclude that to be healthy and happy, people need people, activity, and a purpose. An African word, *ubuntu*, which means "you can't be human alone," expresses our universal need to connect with others. Unfortunately for us, what we need isn't what we get. Studies show that:

- Social isolation and loneliness are common among brain-injury survivors.
- Social isolation increases the risk of sickness, substance abuse, and death, including suicide.
- Community involvement and a sense of purpose or meaning increase feelings of self-worth and enhance quality of life.
- Social interaction strengthens our immune systems so fewer disease-producing organisms can successfully invade our bodies.

How Community Strengthens Immunity

Positive people interactions power us up! When we seek social contacts — such as hugs, high fives, laughter, and love — we find wellness. On the other hand, those who don't interact with others catch sickness. Friends not only fight loneliness, they fight illness!

These human contacts arm our systems — the more numerous and the more varied the better. In their article "Friends can be good medicine," Sobel and Ornstein (1998) found that those with six or more diverse social contacts each day show greater resistance to infection than those with one to three daily contacts. The fewer the social connections in a person's daily life, the greater the chance of illness. Any positive interchange with another human being — however brief — enhances our ability to withstand a viral invasion. *So, smile the next time you see someone!*

How do people help us to avoid bad choices and early death?

When we seek comfort from other people — rather than from things — we are less likely to self-medicate with unhealthy choices in an attempt to heal ourselves.

> Hugs, not drugs!
> — (sign on a bus)

Love heals by its ability to create feelings of self-worth. Love feels good. Love is positive energy. Be sociable — live a long life!

"Who wants to live longer? I want to live better!"

Right! — Me, too! Longevity studies of the general population show that the same qualities that produce life satisfaction — happiness — are the ones that lead to longer lives. Research with survivors shows that life satisfaction after brain injury means leading healthy and productive lives and participating in work and leisure (Corrigan et al., 2001).

By now, most of us know what those healthy behaviors are — commitment to physically and mentally active lifestyles, nutritious eating habits, adequate rest, attendance at religious services, no more than moderate alcohol consumption, no drug use, no tobacco use, and — a social support system.

Social Challenges

What causes survivors' social problems?
Ever notice someone looking at you as if you were nuts because of something you did or said? Me, too! It happens a lot to us! Our social difficulties affect us everywhere we go, from casual encounters to getting — and keeping — a job. As a matter of fact, our social problems cause us more trouble than anything else from our brain injuries.

> You don't live in a world all alone. Your brothers and sisters are here, too.
> — Albert Schweitzer

Why do we act as we do? A social mistake could result from any or all of these: a brain burp (cognitive error), feelings of depression and anxiety, or a behavioral response to our cognitive errors and emotions.

What's the link between mental skills and social activity?
Remember my angry plea *"Fix my brain and I won't be crazy!"*? Researchers found that socially inappropriate behavior was strongly linked to cognitive problems in combat veterans (Prigatano, 1987). Perhaps it went something like this: a soldier returns home from warfare with a bump on the head and can't find his old friend's house. He drives around for a while and notices the neighborhood looks different. Then he telephones his friend and yells, "You moved and you didn't tell me!" Well, nobody moved. The soldier lost his way — and a few other connections — because of his head injury.

Whether we're returning from war or not, we're like that soldier. Is it any surprise then, that the combination of our difficulty remembering and our tendency to say whatever is on our minds creates social problems? Besides having inflexible thinking, we survivors find it difficult to adapt old skills to new situations, to learn from past errors, and — regardless of our intelligence — to adapt to new environments. We may also expect others to think and act the way we do, with predictable — and unhappy — results. With these unseen — but not unnoticed — impairments, we fail — and we fail a lot — personally, socially, and economically.

The good news? As our mental skills improve, so do our social skills! Like other abilities, social skills can be relearned. Just as we regain competence for physical and mental tasks like walking, talking, thinking, and reading, we can relearn how to converse with others and be more socially competent, too.

Keep the faith! This improvement can occur even many years after severe injury! (Thomsen, 1992). So, rather than accept social shortcomings as permanent character defects, work with your therapists to restore previous capacities and skills and to compensate for what was lost — regardless of how long ago you were injured.

Behavioral/Emotional Challenges

"What do you mean? There's nothing wrong with how I act!"

Does this sound like you? Who wants to admit anything is wrong? Refusing to admit problems is common — especially if we don't see them and were fine before the injury. We're furious that we aren't who we were and can't do what we did — or control our emotions. Hell, we can't even identify our feelings, let alone control them! Anger rules us. People avoid us — and who can blame them?

We behave as we feel. The worse we feel, the worse we act. If we realize we are angry and deal with it appropriately when we're with others or excuse ourselves from their company to defuse our anger in a healthy way, our social desirability increases greatly. We must work to fix our social skills if we want to get along with people and have friends.

Personal experience. *Anger is my default emotion, so it reappeared frequently — and without warning — on my long and protracted 30-plus-year journey to acceptance.*

I'm not angry anymore. Sure, I become enraged — perhaps out of proportion — at injustices, but I'm not a constant rager. What happened? People appeared when I needed them.

Anger reduction started with my first good therapist, whom I met at a psychosomatic clinic in El Paso, Texas, where I went because of ulcer pain. DJ, as I call him, a psychologist associated with University Health Services, correctly assessed me as a red-hot cyclone. He allowed me to vent my rage and engaged me cognitively so that I kept coming back for therapy, partly out of curiosity and partly because he met me where I was. He actually walked with me out of the clinic after one of our early sessions, talking to me like a real person, rather than a doctor's patient. When DJ baited me, I threw things — never at him, he pointed out — but I threw things, nonetheless. He knew that I needed to release this overwhelming anger, so didn't remind me that I was nearly 30 years old and adults don't throw things. I especially cherish that he believed I had sustained brain damage, despite the lack of test results to prove it. Finally, someone believed me that something was wrong with my brain!

What are social skills?

Social competence means knowing social rules, reading social cues, and acting appropriately. See *Brain Injury Rewiring for Loved Ones* Chapter 11 for a discussion of the many social skill deficits we're likely to exhibit — if you dare! To summarize, these behaviors include being self-centered, acting impulsively with impatience and irritability, and losing our temper. Environmentally, anything that comes into our space without permission, especially flashing lights or loud noises, is seen as an invader. Before we all just quit and crawl into our caves with our booze, burgers and fries, cigarettes, and video games, let's assume that nobody exhibits all of these behaviors at the same time — *at least I don't think anyone does...*

How does social inadequacy look?
We can divide our social problems into two polar-opposite categories —
too much and too little (Baser, 1998). Let's picture two survivors,
Tommy and Suzy. Although both of their brains were damaged, each
injury is different. Even though they both may lack self-confidence, they
act in opposite ways. One acts out and one acts in.

Differences Too-Much-Tommy acts childlike, is impulsive, impatient, irritable, preoccupied with sex, and talks too much and too loudly.
Tommy may feel everyone is his friend. In contrast, Sad-Suzy, Ms. Too-
Little, doesn't respond to others, acts uncertain, unmotivated, and
inadequate. She is sexually disinterested. Suzy whispers or may not talk
at all. Suzy may feel no one is her friend.

Similarities. They're both out of balance, act inappropriately, and
don't fit socially. While Tommy is over-wired and Suzy is under-wired,
both of them seem self-centered and insensitive to others. Both fail to
learn from their mistakes and don't monitor and correct their behavior.
Even though they act differently, the cause for their behavior is the same.
Unique to us, this behavior is often called the *frontal-lobe personality*
because of the damage to the front of our brains. Like Tommy and Suzy,
we survivors may differ from each another in the ways we act, but we all
share the same basic problem: social inadequacy. Let's learn the cause.

Which cognitive deficits interfere with social skills?
Our numerous deficits make relationships a challenge for one and all.
The most obvious — to others — and the most disabling — to us — is
what is called our *executive function* impairment. When our brain-boss
was injured, our seeing-wires lost solid connections with our thinking-
wires, reducing our abilities to direct and control our behavior.

Socially successful people in all walks of life are good at this multi-
tasking skill. Their brain-boss plans and controls all their interactions and
observes and responds to non-verbal cues. Most survivors can't see this
deficit, which is one reason it is so disabling. We're unaware of the
problem that we need to fix!

This doesn't mean we can't communicate with others. But, to regain
our conversational abilities requires that we work on the impaired steps,
perhaps with a talking coach, and then practice with friends and family.

Gradually, the social interaction process becomes easier and easier, like everything else — if we keep at it. Practice improves performance.

Turn-taking in conversation is an example. To truly respond to a speaker appropriately — rather than just talk — is an art. We need to look, listen, and pay attention to body language before we speak. This complex process of conversation is one that continually challenges many of us, regardless of how long ago our injuries happened. *I continue to work on this after 30 years, but I've improved! Keep the faith!*

Automatic versus manual transmission. For non-injured people, the entire communication process works rapidly and smoothly, similar to an automatic transmission in a car. Survivors, however, now have manual transmissions, so choosing the right gear requires that we analyze the situation before we respond. And with others waiting for us, we need to do this fast — and fast is not one of our speeds! We don't do well when rushed!

Understand that your social skills may never be automatic again. They can, however, flow easier. Just like the phone call between Denver and New York that now needs to go through Chicago — it may not be smooth or fast, but it can happen!

Problem: Missed Cues

Okay, let's face it, sometimes — often? — we just don't act appropriately. Subtleties elude us! Many of us get in trouble because we either don't read body language at all or read it incorrectly. In other words, we don't see and read cues. Whether our inappropriate behaviors are a direct result of our brain injury or in response to it, these deficits are present nonetheless. Denying them doesn't make them go away anymore than ignoring them does! Why are we socially awkward?

Difficulty controlling strong emotions such as anger is common. It is also socially undesirable. Research found inverse (opposite) relationships between anger and forgiveness and between anger and social desirability (Gisi, 2000). *What a surprise!*

Personal experience. *Thanks to good therapy and good friends between 1976 and today, my victim personality remains in my past. Although victim laments like "Why me?" are now occasionally replaced* *by warrior cries of "Bring it on!" at least now I don't watch what happened or wonder what happened — I make things happen!*

The clueless and self-critical survivor whose quote began this chapter changed. Now when communication errors occur — as they unfortunately probably always will — l still look first to my behavior — with one big difference — I seek an error to correct, rather than a fault to criticize.

Sometimes I remember Dr. Baser's wise counsel: "Carolyn, you are not to blame for everything that goes wrong. It may be the other person. Perhaps someone is having a bad day. Perhaps it is their deficit and not yours. Perhaps it is just a breakdown — and no one's fault." Imagine that!

SAFER

Again, a good way to analyze and correct social errors is the SAFER method.

- **Stop.** To see social missteps or errors, we need to be aware and acknowledge that something is wrong.
- **Assess.** Identify what is wrong and understand why it's important to correct errors. Observe your audience for signs that you've lost them: Do others look confused and/or disinterested? Do they look away or appear tired? Is their only response "uh-huh," "Right," etc.?
- **Fix.** Learn ways to repair the miscues. Maybe say, "I'm sorry. I'll try to be more sensitive to your feelings next time. What's a better way to say what I said?" *This approach invites another to help you be a friend. Most people will appreciate your effort and forgive you. If they won't, forget them!*

If it's poor memory that causes you to forget dates and appear unreliable, then use a calendar, day-planner, mini-tape recorder, PDA, Blackberry, etc. to remember those dates.

- **Evaluate.** Assess whether your repair worked. Perhaps ask a socially savvy friend for help. Maybe your inability to recognize social cues causes unsatisfactory social interactions. Then your task is to relearn how to read and understand the cues!

- **Retry.** Find places and times to use your new repertoire of behaviors. Practice social skills just like other skills.

How can the same plan work for everyone?
We're not alike, but we all experience social difficulties, whether our behavior differs from Tommy's and Suzy's a little or a lot.

SAFER works because it's simple — we look at a behavior that can be changed rather than a trait that cannot. SAFER works because it is optimistic. If we look at our current state as dynamic rather than permanent, we can hope rather than despair about our social future. SAFER works because it's fail-proof! If we try something and it doesn't work, we simply retry. And, maybe the next time we ask one of our coaches for help. We can all benefit from our SAFER approach. *I promise!*

Relationship Changes

Marriage and Other Love Partnerships

Your pre-injury love relationship is history. It is not necessarily over, but it is forever changed. If it is strong enough — and able to adapt to your changes — it can reinvent itself. You will certainly mourn the loss of the marriage as it was, but the marriage isn't necessarily over. It can be recreated — with a lot of work from you, your lover, and counselors.

> Love is patient;
> love is kind;
> love is not envious or boastful or arrogant or rude.
> It does not insist on its own way;
> it is not irritable or resentful...
> it bears all things,
> believes all things,
> hopes all things,
> endures all things.
>   — I Corinthians: 13

Personal experience. I initially concluded that brain injury didn't play a role in my failed marriage because we divorced the year before my life-altering car crash. My opinion changed, however, when I thought about two earlier whiplash injuries. Although not considered brain injuries in 1974, obviously something caused head and neck pain! Sufficient damage warranted injections, rehab, medications, and braces.

While I don't remember much, I recall the loss of both my easy-going disposition and a sense of control. I remember sleeping on the couch one Friday after a week of teaching school to avoid awakening my husband with my moaning. (I also feared he'd minimize the pain and refuse to take me to the doctor the next day, so I drove myself).

Was the marriage already in trouble? It's hard to know all these years later what caused the demise of that five-year union, but my behavior certainly changed after those whiplash injuries, and with that, my role in the marriage. Pain does that.

I also recall that my previous healthy lifestyle dissolved in the Valium-booze-water mixes that I began to favor — even developing a fondness for Scotch! While I continued to teach — what, I don't know — medicating the pain wrested the focus of my life away from all other interests. Was this the beginning of the downward spiral?

How can your post-injury marriage reinvent itself?
Recent research concluded that you and your partner need to develop problem-solving strategies that include a positive attitude both toward each other and the difficulty, and facing rather than avoiding problems (Blais & Boisvert, 2007). With help, you can learn or relearn these skills!

How many of us live in a love relationship?
The percentages of married or cohabiting heterosexuals varied from 34% of 454 Canadian survivors 13 years post-injury (Dawson & Chipman, 1995) to 75% of 120 American survivors of all brain injury categories between two and one-half and eight years after injury (Kreutzer et al., 2007). Swedish researchers found 58% of 92 survivors enjoyed a stable relationship. Encouragingly, 55% of these relationships began after injury (Kreuter et al., 1998). This shows that post-injury love can happen!

Pre-Injury Friendships

The chief reason friendships die is usually the lost link between you and your friend(s). It's no one's fault, really. With no connection, there are no sparks, so the relationship doesn't work anymore. Here's a possible scenario: pre-injury, every week a group of you played ball and then went to a bar to socialize. If you are no longer able to play, don't want to coach or watch, and that was the only link, the friendships die. Your former teammates' lives didn't change and their former friend is now a stranger, so they don't seek you out or return your calls.

Avoidance is a typical response for many other reasons. Some friends may fear that other people will look at them as if they're brain-injured, too. Can we blame them if they avoid damaged goods? Or maybe being with you makes them feel at risk: "If it happened to him, it could happen to me, too, so I'd better stay away." Others may try to deny that the injury ever happened. If they stay away, both of you can avoid the pain of remembering how good it used to be. Perhaps they feel awkward around you and don't know what to do or say. Another reason to avoid you is simple but painful — there's no reason to be with you. Whatever you used to do together is no longer an option. You just don't fit. No more mutual esteem. No more fun. No more friendship.

We survivors need to try to not be angry with those who simply are not strong enough — or interested enough — to remain in a relationship. We can be very demanding, and other peoples' needs may frequently be overlooked. Unless they're saints and we're a "cause," they'll find other friends. Consider that what people say and do reflects and reveals who they are, as well as their relationship with us. Maybe it's their deficit and not ours!

Can we be friends again? Yes. As our self-centeredness gradually diminishes, others may be able to relax and enjoy being with us. As we rewire, our friends may not always have to place our needs first — their needs can be considered, too, so it's more of a mutual friendship.

And as the years pass, it is possible that some old friends may return. *Thankfully, I can say this happens!* It is also possible that they may not. All we can do is to be the best we can be; we will attract others into our lives who didn't know us before — and who like us now! *Some new friends may not have been attracted to us before our injury, either — amazingly enough!*

Post-Injury Friendships

Making friends post-injury is just like it was before — those with mutual needs or interests connect or an indefinable spark occurs. And, just like with pre-injury friends, the friendship dies if any of those things change or are lost.

Keeping friends is different now. Sometimes it's about us, sometimes it's about them, and sometimes it's both. In the strange-but-true category, our progress can actually cause problems! If we continue to grow and to develop and they don't, the one-sided growth can jeopardize the friendship. Some friends may be threatened by these changes and choose to end the relationship; others may be unable to keep pace with us — isn't that a switch! Those who encourage growth are the kinds of friends that we will keep and cherish.

Some people we first attract post-injury may need to keep a teacher-student (giver-taker) type of relationship in order to maintain the friendship. Again, if they need us to remain the same, it demonstrates their inadequacy — not ours. And, while we lose their mentoring, they lose, too. As we all know, uneven relationships don't usually last, unless the needs of both are met. Some people need to be needed, and when they perceive they are not, they seek another person in distress. Another sad loss — but it is a sign that we are growing and leaving one of our cocoons. While growth is often painful, we need to remember that it is also good. As we grow, we not only feel less inadequate — we are!

Situations where it's more about us include those times when we commit a social error. While new friends may initially overlook it or laugh about it, if we continue to act inappropriately, it could become awkward for them to continue to associate with us.

Another "more about us" possibility is that the intensity that initially attracted them may become more than they want to deal with on a regular basis, so they end the relationship. If they refuse to talk about it, we won't know what we did, which may or may not be anything specific — maybe it's just that we're red-hot now and they're mellow-yellow!

Remember, some people may not like our sparks! And, as always, we can only be responsible for our own attitudes and actions — it's impossible to control the attitudes and actions of others. Trying to do so makes us unhappy and rarely changes others for the better, anyway! So, go where people like sparks! If they only want to put out the fire, we'd probably eventually decide we didn't want to be around them, either!

Relationship changes also may relate less to disability and more to human nature. People mature and grow in different directions. As interests change and new attractions replace old ones, the common bond is lost. It's not a bad thing — it just happens. Either new connections develop or the friendship is over. Just remember — it was good when it was good.

Strategies for Friendship

After our injury, a lot of losses occurred. If we just sit around alone and brood, not only will we lose more, but the light that attracts people into our sphere will diminish or vanish, too. What can we do? Many ideas are included in lists at the end of this chapter, but for now, consider these:

> And let there be no purpose in friendship save the deepening of the spirit...
> — Kahlil Gibran

- **Visit someone worse off than you.** People in nursing homes and rehab centers are usually very receptive. You may find someone who can provide that unconditional love you need — and you may find someone who can help you in your recovery beyond just being receptive. They may need a friend, too, so it could be another win-win situation.
- **Acknowledge that you are not the same.** And perhaps even joke about it to ease the discomfort of others. This is a good example of how a memorial service could increase everyone's awareness and reduce awkwardness. See Chapter 6 "Emotional Rewiring."
- **Understand that your friends may not be able to accept** your need to manage your environment, considering it too controlling. If they value you as a friend, they will accept it as part of who you are. If not, you don't need their friendship!
- **Accept that we can be very needy,** so allow your friends to set some of the parameters of the friendship. For example: rather than

calling them on your time frame, agree on a mutual time to talk or ask, "Is this a good time to talk?"

Former Relationships with Drinking and/or Drugs

"Okay, lady. I understand the common-bond thing. But what if the connection was drinking or doing drugs? That's what we did! Now, if I use I damage myself even more. What's up, now?"

> There can be no Friendship where there is no Freedom.
> — William Penn

Think SAFER — Stop. Assess the situation. Fix it. In this case, the "F" also stands for "Find," like find new activities, find new friends. Don't like those ideas? Then how about find new interests and activities with your current friends?

"Yeah, right. Like my buddies are gonna wanna go to church to meet girls!"

Not a bad idea, actually. Typically, more women attend religious services than guys. The point is to be proactive rather than reactive. What this means is that you suggest ideas rather than wait for your friends to "forget" to pick you up a few times. Not to blame anyone. It's human nature to keep doing what we're doing because it's comfortable and it works — until it doesn't work.

Obviously, drinking with your buddies doesn't work anymore if it led to the brain injury. Even if it didn't, the odds are that next time it will, what with 60% of all TBIs being substance-related (Corrigan et al., 1995). And now, post-injury, you can expect a "go to jail" card. Because of our lack of control, what happens now is drink, drug, fight, get arrested. Many TBI survivors who are arrested are classified as "aggressive." And a recent study found a high incidence of heavy drinking — both pre- and post-injury — among patients with an arrest history (Kreutzer et al., 1995). Do you see a link here? See Chapter 6 "Emotional Rewiring" to refresh your memory about the health dangers of post-injury alcohol and drug use.

Dating

Is dating now any different from dating before injury? Well, yes, it is. Now, in addition to the vulnerabilities of dating, we can add the complexities of disability. Do we say: "Oh goody, I love a challenge!" Or not?

Well, fellow survivors, that's the way it is. If we choose to date, then we date with a disability. If our disability hampers us — and to what degree — only we can decide. We can view dating as another skill to rewire and add practice to our SAFER procedure — Stop, Assess, Fix, Evaluate, Retry. Or we can sit home with the TV, video games, computer, or book and rotate these "dates" of choice. What sounds more appealing and healthier? *Hint: social isolation leads to more depression.*

Aren't the reasons for dating the same as pre-injury: enjoyment, companionship, sexual attraction, and maybe finding a life/marriage partner? It is not something we must do. It is something we choose to do — when we're ready.

You may ask, "Will anyone want me?" It depends — are you attractive to others? Getting ready to date is like preparing for a job interview. In both cases, we want to look our best, right? So ask yourself "Do I look like I am friends with the shower and the barber? Are my clothes neat and clean?" And, if you smoke, maybe wait to see if your date smokes because others may not want to kiss an ashtray — or smell one.

Why would anyone choose your company? Do you like yourself — and others? Do you care about anything beyond yourself? Are you fun to be with, interesting, and kind? Are you passionate about life and/or any causes? What are your interests and long-term goals? Your desirability is probably related more to who you are than what you look like.

Remember, it's our behavior that causes social problems, so seek help for deficit areas such as anger. You can do it! The more we socialize, the better we get — the more we stay alone, the worse we get!

How do you know if you're ready to date? Ask people you trust. In addition to family and friends, seek the counsel of others in various social circles, perhaps a support or religious group. If they're vague, ask what you need to do to be ready. Then, work on those areas!

How successful are survivors in finding compatible soul mates?
Injury is not a major barrier to love! Research finds that many survivors
are single, do not socialize as much as they did before their injury, and
are not involved in a romantic relationship (Burton et al., 2003, among
others). Still, meeting someone compatible can happen! In fact, a study
in Sweden of 92 survivors, age range of 20-70 with a median age-at-
injury of 32, found that 58% of them enjoyed a stable relationship and
55% of these relationships were established post-injury! (Kreuter et al.,
1998).

How do I meet compatible people to date?
Here's one area with increased options post-injury! Now you can add
disability groups for socializing, too! And, just as pre-injury, you can
take a class in an academic interest or physical area, join a health club,
attend a place of worship, go to clubs, or go to an event (concert, play,
lecture, race, game). Seek out activities that interest you and explore
stores that focus on these areas — animals, computers, cars, cooking,
photography, fitness, sports, etc. Many groups advertise their meetings in
the local papers or on line — a recent list offered over 60 activities! If
you think "spiritual connections" to meet others, whether places of
worship or yoga classes, you're in luck!

You can also ask friends to introduce you to others and respond to
and/or place personal ads — in newspapers or on the Internet. How
effective are these "seek-a-date" opportunities? It depends on your goals.
They probably work as well as they did pre-injury. *I don't know. I didn't
do them before. Now I've done all of these in many variations! (And
that's another story…)*

My survivor-tips for dating and social activities:
- Be prepared! Consider and rehearse answers to inevitable questions
  like "Why is someone so attractive, smart, educated, well-dressed,
  etc. alone?", "What are you doing with a handicapped sticker?",
  "What do you do all day?", "Do you work?"
- Just because someone asks a question doesn't mean you're required
  to answer it in any lengthy manner — especially not with a blow-by-

blow history of the injury, hospital stay, etc.! A social encounter is not a doctor's appointment or a legal proceeding.

- If you choose to respond, your answer can be lighthearted, serious, or a combination of these — depending on your mood and the setting (date, casual gathering, etc.). For example: if someone asks, "Why isn't someone so…married?" one reply is "I wasn't suitable for many years — and now I am." You can add a flirtatious remark like "So look out!" — if you're attracted to the questioner. And, with a good retort, you make use that old football adage, "the best defense is a good offense."

- If you give a serious reply, answer and then switch the focus to the other person — ask them a question — or to another topic of mutual interest, like the weather, current and local events, etc. Why dwell on the negative?

- Ask questions that require more than a one-word answer. For example: "What did you do last weekend?", "What are your interests, favorite sports…?", "Do you follow any teams?", "What's one of your all-time favorite movies?" Follow up with "Why?" If someone expresses an interest in computers, maybe ask, "How could my computer work better?"

- Ask opinion questions. For example: "Why do you think New Year's resolutions are so difficult for people to keep?", "Who's going to win the …?" Ask about any current topic of interest — politics, sports event, entertainment, etc. Many options await you!

- Compliment someone about their appearance and then ask where they shop, get their hair done, etc.

Personal experience. *When DJ told me, "You've got to kiss a lot of toads to find a prince," my first response was, "How many toads do I need to kiss? Please don't tell me it's 'as many as it takes!'"*

Sex

As with many other functions that people take for granted until injury, sexual and reproductive functions can be severely disturbed after TBI (Zasler & Horn, 1990).

But wait — there's hope! While sexual dysfunction among survivors is common, only two areas are markedly different from those pre-injury: orgasm and drive/desire (Sandel et al., 1996). *Isn't one enough?*

Since our whole being is involved in the sexual act, everything needs to work. If it doesn't, we need to learn why. When all parts of sexual behavior are assessed — whether neuromedical, behavioral, or psychological — and information is available to your treatment team, you can learn how to treat your dysfunction. Treatment options may include education, counseling, exercise, medications, and/or adaptive equipment.

What physical factors are affected?
As with most aspects of TBI, individuals vary. Different kinds of injuries produce different kinds of damage, both seen and unseen. In addition to the invisible neurological and hormonal factors, many visible conditions play a role in a satisfactory sexual experience, both at genital and nongenital levels. Post-injury male genital dysfunction may include problems with erection, ejaculation, and orgasm. Female dysfunction may involve problems with libido, vaginal lubrication, and orgasm.

At a nongenital level for both genders, range of motion around major joints and other sensory, motor, and physical capabilities, as well as bowel and bladder control, affect both sexual positioning and expression.

Affecting both genital and nongenital areas is endocrine dysfunction, which often accompanies TBI, and which needs evaluation because hormones contribute to sexual functioning. Any of a number of imbalances can impact the functioning of various hormones, from thyroid to testosterone. Additionally, other physical injuries and diseases, as well as medications for those conditions, may interfere not just with hormonal function — but with the diagnostic testing (Zasler & Horn, 1990).

Lifestyle factors such as stress, sleep, and exercise also contribute to both the dysfunction and the mystery of sex. And remember that grooming and hygiene play an important role in both attraction and sexual expression as well — no differently than pre-injury. (*Just because the organ works doesn't mean sex occurs.*)

Does the injury site relate to the degree of satisfaction? Good news for frontal-lobe survivors! While we know that exaggeration is common in this group, recent research notes that those who sustained a frontal lobe lesion reported overall higher levels of sexual satisfaction and functioning than those survivors without this type of injury. *And we thought frontal-lobe injuries were all bad!* Survivors of right-hemisphere injuries also reported higher levels of both sexual arousal and experiences (Sandel et al., 1996).

What happens to our sexual desire?
As with many traits, we have either "too much or too little." Those with an increase in desire may exhibit what is called hypersexual or disinhibited sexual behavior. A decreased sex drive is called hyposexuality — survivors demonstrate sexual disinterest or indifference. Although both of these behaviors may illustrate preoccupation or lack of control, their physical basis and treatments differ. Medications directed at the cause are used to control each of these sexually inappropriate behaviors (Zasler & Horn, 1990).

Why does sexual interest change?
A brain injury commonly changes libido (sexual drive and desire) — and you probably know by now in which direction yours went! Research documents that hyposexuality is far more likely to occur than hypersexuality — *while this keeps us out of trouble, it also keeps us out of bed!*

Many factors can decrease sex drive, so before you seek treatment for a physical dysfunction, first consider the various psychological and mental factors that affect sexuality for everyone — whether injured or not.

Hyposexuality can be the result of any or a combination of the following: cognitive dysfunction, organic affective disorders (manic or depressed mood), a generalized reactive depression to the injury, stress and anxiety about body image, feelings of inadequacy, and loss of self-esteem. Other factors that can affect libido include sensitivity to alcohol and to certain medications, depending on the dosage/amount and duration of use/treatment (Zasler & Horn, 1990).

A treatment plan depends on the diagnosis and may include activating antidepressants and hormonal supplementation. Of course, if "it's all in your head," then the treatment plan likely will include a different kind of sex therapy, such as counseling, education, training, — a change of partners? Any number of possibilities! (Zasler & Horn, 1990).

What male genital dysfunctions may occur after a brain injury?
Dysfunction may include problems with erections, ejaculations, and orgasm — no different from pre-injury. The first place to look is at medications. Some medications that survivors may take can impair erectile function, lower ejaculation threshold, or lower libido. (*Not all at the same time, thankfully — just one is enough!*) Frequently, loss of sensation is a direct result of diabetes mellitus or long-term tobacco, alcohol, or chronic recreational drug use — *another reason not to smoke or use drugs!* Poor nutrition and lack of exercise also play a part. Other causes of erection difficulties are the many sensory and motor deficits that accompany TBI (Zasler & Horn, 1990).

What are the treatment options for impotence?
There are currently three ways to treat erectile dysfunction (ED): oral (like Viagra and similar medications) or injected medication, penile implants, and external devices. In plain English, this means you can swallow, inject, insert, add, or wear "an assistant" to achieve sexual function.

For those who desire a physical addition, popular surgical methods are penile implants or prostheses — either inflatable or non-inflatable devices. Certain cognitive and physical attributes are necessary for their success (*like the ability to think and blow simultaneously*), but numerous studies of recipients without brain injuries have shown high satisfaction.

External devices such as vacuum pumps are becoming more popular. Compared to other interventions, pumps are preferred for their low cost, safety, and their non-surgical nature (Zasler & Horn, 1990; Zasler, 1992).

For those who experience sexual dysfunction from their SSRI medication, a recent study found that 88% reported improvement after adding a low dose of another medication like mianserin or bupropion to their regimen — with minimal side effects (Dolberg et al., 2002).

Other ways to apply the erection-inducing prostaglandin medication are also available. One system uses a device to insert a suppository; another uses a gel that's rubbed on (Goldstein, 1996). *That sounds like fun!*

Alternative ways to treat impotence include homeopathy and naturopathy, Chinese herbs and supplements, and non-synthetic alternatives to Viagra such as Vialafill (an oral source of nitric oxide, a vasodilator that increases blood flow).

What are treatment options for female genital dysfunction?
Little research regarding female sexual problems after brain injury is available, although it is likely that similar neurological disorders and orthopedic, motor, and sensory deficits affect both sexes. Medications may affect women differently, however, and they may experience difficulties with vaginal lubrication due to the drying effects of various chemical agents.

The same treatments that menopausal women use can work for female survivors: oral and implanted medications (either homeopathic or artificial), Chinese medicine, artificial lubrication, external devices/sex toys, and an uninhibited partner (Zasler & Horn, 1990). Experiment!

If SSRIs reduce your libido, taking a low dose of medication like mianserin or bupropion to combat this side effect can be helpful. Other treatment options to increase sexual desire include topical application of hormonal creams (testosterone and/or estrogen). Increasing blood flow to the vaginal tissues with prostaglandin cream is also effective. Ask your doctor!

How can bowel and bladder problems be treated?
Here's another opportunity for partners to practice acceptance and creativity! Due to the prevalence of frontal lobe injury among TBI survivors, bowel and bladder disturbances are common. Those that can interfere with sexuality include urinary urgency, incontinence (leaking), and altered bowel habits, including the need for use of an ostomy bag.

Changes in these functions don't necessarily eliminate sexual expression in and of themselves. As with most aspects of brain injury, it is how the change is managed by the survivor — and, of course, the survivor's partner — that makes the difference. It may be "all in the timing." For example: you can plan sexual activity around toilet schedules, you can alter food and fluid intake, and you can learn about positioning of catheters and ostomy bags for optimal sexual expression (Zasler & Horn, 1990).

How can we manage cognitive and behavioral problems?

Sexual functioning is significantly affected by these changes. However — whatever the problems — numerous effective treatment options await our personal clinical investigation!

Okay, so maybe using a pager to remind us that it's time for sex isn't our first choice! Other strategies are available to manage the changes that impair our full sexual expression. These interventions, similar to those for physical factors, include medications, counseling, and behavioral modification. Traditional medications like hormones, stimulants, antidepressants, lithium, or anticonvulsants may be prescribed; atypical drugs like beta-blockers, calcium-channel blockers, or amino acids may also be used (Zasler & Horn, 1990). Once again, think SAFER to test a variety of approaches. *After all, maybe the pager would work as a memory tool!*

Sexual satisfaction

On the good-news side, no relationship exists between level of sexual activity and level of physical disability, cognitive impairment, or length of post-traumatic amnesia (Zasler & Kreutzer, 1991).

As for not-so-good news, sexual dysfunction after brain injury is common. As discussed, sexual problems include a decrease in sex drive for both genders as well as a decrease in male erectile function, leading to a reduced frequency of intercourse. Decreases in libido correlate with injury severity. Interestingly, no relationship was found between location of injury and presence of sexual dysfunction, although there was a sharp reduction in sexual activity (Zasler & Kreutzer, 1991).

Time since injury does play an important role, however, with the newbies reporting greater levels of sexual arousal than those not recently injured (Sandel et al., 1996). *Survivors, why is this? Is it due to easier arousal and younger age for those recently injured or is it depression, loss of social contacts, or cumulative losses for long-termers — or a combination? Please comment on my blog at* www.rewiring.org.

As with all other areas of concern to us, when a fulfilling sex life is one of the losses of brain injury, counseling can come to the rescue! Both genders can learn alternative techniques and use adaptive devices. *In other word, don't let the fear of striking out get in your way!*

Relearning Social Skills

What is social competence?

Social competence includes showing interest in another — which may or may not be easy. After a trauma, people are very egocentric — and need to be, to recover. Unfortunately, this self-centeredness continues to a greater or

> All conversations are a dance where you're trying to get in step to a shared rhythm.
> — Diane Rennell, PhD

lesser degree for a very long time. On the other hand, if someone's objective is to pay attention to another, he can remain relaxed because his goal is to focus on the other, which is what social ease is all about.

As part of our rewiring process, we need to put our manual transmission in the correct gear to drive smoothly. Like it or not, we know that most former automatic behaviors departed when our injuries arrived. Like other losses, we may fondly recall their former presence — yet find them only in our daydreams. So if we want to become more socially competent, we need to intentionally relearn social skills.

We can set ourselves up for success if we analyze which activities and people will bring us the most joy. Here's a strategy to learn if a setting is a good place to practice social skills training:

- Draw a target shape with five rings.
- Place favorite activities and people in the inner rings.
- Place acceptable activities and people in outer rings.
- Do not include unpredictable activities or marginal people — avoid the stress of potentially negative experiences.

How to use targets to prepare for interactions:

- Evaluate where a person/activity is located on your target.

- At first, do activities only with inner-ring people.
- With confidence, gradually include outer-ring people and activities to broaden horizons and test skills.

For example, when Too-Much-Tommy sees a waitress, he mentally places her in the outer ring, and doesn't kiss her hand! However, Sad-Suzy might insert a compliment or small talk about the weather into the order/conversation — if the waitress doesn't appear hurried! This approach is based on the technique of progressive desensitization often used with those who have post-traumatic stress disorder (PTSD). First, they do the least stressful things accompanied by a coach, then gradually more difficult things with a coach, and finally they do everything alone.

Where to practice:
- **Therapy settings.** Use such safe settings to draw your targets of people, places, and activities. Subsequent sessions can review experiences in different rings and explore how to increase successful interactions.
- **Real-world settings.** Choose people-friendly places.

Personal experience. Friends who are especially kind and coura-geous can provide helpful hints. Here's an example: In the early 1980s — when I was really bad!! — a friend from Christ Presbyterian Church of La Costa frequently provided on-the-spot analyses and tips like "another way to say that would be..." This was especially important when she overheard a conversational mistake that I made or when I was confused by something someone said. She also noticed that my eyes darted back and forth when someone asked me a question that momentarily baffled me. Thanks to her, I can now tell others that my brain scrolls like a computer when it searches for the correct answer in its library. Jane was available to call on at any time — and her willingness to share some of her diplomatic secrets is still appreciated and used. Find your special friends who care enough to really help — especially when you're clueless about "how do I respond to that?"

- **Religious settings** can be welcoming and forgiving, and offer opportunities to both give and receive. These can be good places for us because reaching out to others in need is typically a mission. Also, worshippers are often aware of their own imperfections, so they are quite likely to accept others who exhibit faults.

Personal experience. I really found my niche as a greeter for newcomers when my friend, Kay Armstrong, asked me to join the Welcome Ministry. It especially suits me because my services are needed every Sunday, providing lots of practice!

- **Community social service agencies** also present forgiving practice settings, especially for volunteers. Other workers are generally passionate about their cause and overlook personal quirks, and recipients are generally glad for your help! Health-care settings are usually effective because they're familiar — we can relax and people can see our best selves, making the experience good for all. Ushering at arts events and helping at sports events gives us lots of practice, too. See Chapter 12 for other ideas and the end of this chapter for more examples.

Personal experience. As a low-income performing-arts lover, ushering at cultural events provides a free way for me to enjoy theater, symphony, and various concerts that are beyond my necessities-only budget. The vast majority of these experiences are delightful! Not only is practice of social skills always available, once I was in the power-position as a hostess of the event and another time I "gonged" the intermission at a symphony concert! Fun!

What can we do to improve our social skills?
- Acknowledge that something is wrong.
- Work to fix it. Observe and copy those you admire, ask for tips, and then apply your learning.
- Practice — practice — practice! Practice in therapy, in comfortable and forgiving settings, and with agreeable friends.
- Fake it till you make it.
- Rely on God/religious family, personal drive, friends, family, and other helpers.

- Follow the SAFER formula (Stop, Assess, Fix, Evaluate, Retry). Who knows, some day you may occasionally feel socially at ease in some unfriendly real-world settings. It could happen! And remember — small steps for success!

People often feel their load is heavier, their mountain is higher, their air is thinner, their body is weaker. Doesn't everyone carry a loaded backpack — whether visibly injured or not? Burdens that others carry may not be obvious. For example, many people with diabetes, cancer, asthma, and hearing disorders look "normal." Also, consider those with "heart" conditions — whether physical or emotional. While some people may carry a heavy heart, others' hearts are hardened from injury, hurt, and neglect. Small hearts are not visible either, yet we all know what it feels like to be around one and may label him/her as a Grinch or a Scrooge.

Personal experience. I'm gradually learning to remind myself that problems are not always personal, pervasive, or permanent (the three bad Ps). Life is not black or white, but usually some shade of gray. Think how wise I'll be when I'm older!

Setting Goals for Social Skills Relearning

To make oneself understood is usually considered a reasonable goal for everyone. For survivors, something else may be equally as important.

Personal experience. My dear friend, Patricia Marshall, a former president of the San Diego Brain Injury Foundation, courageously asked me once, "Could one of your goals just be smooth conversation?"

First, I insisted, "No way! I need to be understood." Later, I decided that perhaps "smooth conversation" is a worthy goal because if all we do is try to make everyone understand us, who will want to be our friends? Survivors can often be accused — and rightly so — of being broadcasters, not receivers. Why should anyone else want to listen to us if we don't want to listen to them? This broadcaster concept can be difficult for survivors to grasp; it will remain a problem until we decide to show at least as much interest in others' opinions as in our own. We may just learn something! My lifesaver psychologist, DJ, first proposed the broadcaster concept to me — I didn't understand it for about 10 years!

Strategies and Aids for Survivors

- If you feel overloaded, leave the situation or ask for help.
- Request conversation-partners to ask only one question at a time, especially if you're overloaded.
- Use external aids (date book, calendar, PDAs, etc.) to record information (appointments, tasks) if memory is a problem.
- Read nametags to reinforce name and face recognition.
- Show interest with eye contact, enthusiasm, and body posture.
- Repeat someone's name during the conversation to connect it with his or her face. Maybe create a rhyming word for the name.
- Remember that respect, graciousness, and friendliness can overcome most social offenses.
- Confess to a memory goof with an apology. "I'm sorry, I don't remember. What is your name again?" usually works.
- Ask someone else for help if you forget a name. This creates a win-win situation.
- Observe the behavior of those you admire and ask them for tips later. This is a compliment!
- If appropriate, suggest using a game to remember names.
- Ask other group members to display name cards or tags.
- In group settings where people are seated, make a chart of peoples' names. *I love to use this memory technique because when I use it people always marvel at how smart I am — rather than ask what's wrong with my memory!*
- "Fake it til you make it." To maintain smooth conversation, just smile, nod, or agree.
- Be active in many pursuits.

Personal experience. To aid my social inadequacy I stored responses in my brain that I could call on when stuck. These ready answers were a collection of sayings from people I admired. Watching and listening to these special friends, typically in the social hour after church, gave me a repertoire of acceptable things to say until I could develop my own.

How to Overcome Deficits and Relearn Social Skills

How do we learn/relearn social competence? Think SAFER. Stop and assess social skills, work to fix them, evaluate what you did, and then retry, using different strategies. Because of our jumbled wires, we probably exhibit some social skills and lack others. With our manual transmission, we need specific input. Generally, the best programs use a step-by-step approach and practice various skills in real-life situations. See *Brain Injury Rewiring for Loved Ones,* Chapter 11, for a longer discussion of two effective programs.

Developing Social Skills (William H. Burke, 1997) is a program that details basic and advanced social skills, suggests a group interaction format, and provides rating scales that can be used. Included are ways to accept feedback — whether criticism or compliments, how to both express and accept an apology, and suggested responses to answer the problematic "What do I say?"

The Conversation Improvement Program (Mark Ylvisaker, 1997) is another "fix my brain and I won't be crazy" approach. Skills that are taught in this approach are those that are generally

> Often the best way to persuade others is with your ears.
> — Dean Rusk

acquired as we grow, but often need to be deliberately retaught to us after our injuries. The program focuses on the different parts of conversation and how to interpret social behavior.

Strategies to Set Ourselves Up for Success

Try the following strategies for more fluid social interactions:
- Interact with six or more people per day by phone or in person.
- Choose social contacts with a high percentage of success — those activities, places, and people in the inner rings of your target.
- Prepare your body, mind, and spirit with sleep, healthy food, and exercise.
- Know where you're going and who'll be there.
- Pay attention to the speaker, maintain eye contact, and ask questions.
- Remember: be a receiver — not just a broadcaster!

- Show interest and enthusiasm in posture and voice — smile, laugh, and nod your head.
- If confused, ask the speaker to repeat information, and then record it.
- Practice and critique conversations with friends: "Did I say that right?", "What's a better way to say…?" Rehearse rules.

Personal experience. *Even after 30 years, reading non-verbal behavior remains challenging, so I tell people I need verbal feedback, which is not always possible. I have come to accept my liability and no longer feel so inadequate. What do I do? I smile, go on, and maybe later ask someone to interpret and explain. Friends know and accept this, and it isn't as much of a problem anymore with them. Strangers, however, are another matter, and that solution is still brewing.*

External Memory Aids

- Day-timer notebook or similar logbook — even better with brain-in-a-binder insert.
- PDA, cell phone, tape recorder.
- Calendars: wall, desk, pocket or purse, and on the computer.
- Sticky notes, note pads and cards, pens and pencils.
- Timers — note the reason for the timed reminder! (J. Hein, 1997, 1998)
- Electronic pagers: *NeuroPage* automatic programmable reminder system (www.neuropage.nhs.uk/).

Real-World Practice

"Seek and ye shall find." This saying applies to many areas, none more so than finding friends. The more we seek them, the better chance we'll find them! And, if we don't seek, we'll never find. For sure, they won't appear out of a television set — no matter how high-tech.

We're ready now to venture forth and test our new skills. We want to be with others and to be involved in our community. We also know that involvement is the first step away from the egocentricity that is inevitable with a traumatic sickness or injury. Got it? Let's go!

Where do we go? It depends on our desired level of involvement: to watch or participate. We'll obviously go only where we're wanted, which guarantees a successful experience. We need to seek social settings where people are more likely to accept atypical behavior and that offer good role models for what is appropriate. The best places offer a high probability of acceptance. Find your bliss!

Survivor and Family/Friends Activities

Share anything of interest that stimulates your brain. Here are some ideas:

> There is no greater desert or wilderness than to be without true friends.
> — Francis Bacon

Quiet

- Talk about your lives now; dream and plan for the future.
- Discuss what you've recently learned from the newspaper, magazines, books, television, radio, computer.
- Watch TV or videos together and discuss what is happening, what it means, what will likely happen next, and what each of you would do if you were the lead character.
- Try the idea above with the sound muted!
- Work on therapy assignments.
- Listen to music or play music together.
- Play/work on the computer and/or surf the net together.

More Active

- Play indoor games with another person (board, card, even computer games if there is useful social interaction).
- Plan and prepare a meal, then clean up.
- Do outdoor tasks and then reward yourselves with play.
- Play active physical games, do outdoor activities or sports.
- Attend a sporting event, fair, or other community event.
- Visit the library, bookstores, art galleries, and museums.
- Attend performing arts events and movies. Discuss what you saw.
- Dine, shop, window-shop, investigate the neighborhood.
- Volunteer at community events.
- Play with a pet.

Activities and groups in the community

Disability-related groups.
Your community probably offers a brain-injury support group through a hospital or college. Offering kinship and social skills practice, as well as helpful information, such groups meet in accessible community

> People do not live together merely to be together. They live together to do something together.
> — Ortega Gasset

areas. Typically, brain injury foundations serve both caregivers and survivors. Some sponsor survivors to attend various seminars and classes.

Non-disability groups.
Of the many reasons to participate in a group with others who may or may not be disabled, perhaps the most important are
- The focus is on ability and not disability.
- We are considered equals because we share an interest.
- Other participants usually act socially appropriately.

Personal experience. I found that groups without a disability focus were the most helpful to me because of these reasons. Keep in mind, too, that when I was injured in 1976 there weren't any appropriate disability-related groups, so I had no choice! Maybe participate in both!

Some Examples of Groups Include:

Theme-related:
- Health-related (brain/spinal cord injury, etc.).
- Support and growth (12-step, divorce, single parents, grief, etc.).

> Grief can take care of itself, but to get the full value of a joy you must have somebody to divide it with.
> — Mark Twain

- Religious. *My fave — these people promise to love one another!*
- Study (book, religious, issue, computer, or school-related).
- Local neighborhood (Neighborhood Watch, etc.).
- Nature/environmental (Sierra Club, etc.).
- Animal — some focus on training pets for others.

- Singles with various emphases (walking, writing, gardening, etc.).
- Youth-related (YMCA, Boys & Girls Clubs, etc.)

Note: With some theme groups, it is better if the group is "closed." This means that nobody joins and nobody quits after a certain time. The advantages are obvious — bonding and accountability. If people know they'll be missed, they'll attend. In mutual-concern groups such as divorce recovery, people share sensitive information.

Activity-related:
- Performing arts groups — music, theater, improv comedy, etc.
- Visual arts, photography, computer, garden.
- Craft/sewing/woodwork/other handwork.
- Computer-user groups & Internet.
- Auto or motorcycle — restoring and operating.
- Model airplane/model car.
- Radio communications.
- Sport/fitness (participate/race); gym/health club.
- Teams (play or coach/assist).
- Indoor games (bridge, puzzles, etc.).
- School, library, or hospital-related.
- Community centers (senior & recreation).
- Volunteer opportunities — local papers and Craig's List on the Internet (www.Craigslist.com) usually list dozens.

Personal experience. Some years ago, a fire swept through a residential area near my former home and left many people homeless. When I attended my first Sunday service at a local church, I learned that it would serve as a distribution center for needed items for those residents who lost everything in the fire. Because as a writer, my schedule was my own, I volunteered to distribute clothing during the day. What happened? I met wonderful people, was useful, enjoyed the contacts, and was even asked to join the chaplaincy program of the agency that sponsored the relief effort! "God moves in mysterious ways!"

How to find groups/clubs/teams:
Go on line, visit stores, check your newspaper (ours listed hundreds!), contact your city recreation department, and explore phonebook Yellow pages. Let your fingers do the walking, then get active!

Summary

Although we may never return to our former social-butterfly days (real or imagined), social rewiring is possible. Keep in mind that what we do — not what we are — causes our social difficulties. Believe that you can make friends again! Some final thoughts:

> Behavior change precedes attitude change.
> — M. Isenhart

- Socialize in friendly places.
- Practice your social skills in therapy and real-world places.
- Choose social interactions with a high chance of success (best activities, places, and people).
- Show interest with eye contact, enthusiasm, and posture.
- Be prepared for questions when you date — and otherwise.
- Just because someone asks a question doesn't mean you're required to answer it in any lengthy manner.
- Ask others "why?", "how?", and opinion questions.
- Remember that the best defense is a good offense.
- Observe behavior of those you admire and ask them for tips.
- Respect, graciousness, and friendliness can overcome most social offenses.
- Be a receiver — not just a broadcaster!
- Fake it till you make it.
- Beware thinking everything involves the Three Ps: personal, pervasive, and permanent.
- Know that there's hope if you have sexual dysfunction after injury.
- If you feel either internally or externally overloaded, leave the situation immediately or ask for help.
- Prepare your body, mind, and spirit for outings with sleep, good nutrition, exercise, readiness.
- Interact with six or more people per day.

- Be active in many pursuits.
- Practice SAFER (Stop, Assess, Fix, Evaluate, Retry).
- Know that you can learn new behaviors — our brains are "plastic."
- Not all social glitches result from our mistakes.
- Open, affirming, and welcoming people and places do exist! Keep searching to find them!

12

Vocational Rewiring: Healing with Productive Activity

How many doors do I have to knock on?
— Carolyn E. Dolen
As many as it takes.
— Psychologist DJ

"Work? Who, me? You've got to be kidding! What can I do? I'm disabled. Besides, I look/talk/speak/move funny. Who'd want me, anyway? Why work? Who needs work to be happy?"

Introduction

We do! Productive activity so positively influences our happiness that nearly 200 survivors stated that employment was the strongest contributor to their improved quality of life (Webb et al., 1995).

Why? People seek activity and meaning in their lives to be happy. If we feel a sense of purpose, we won't need to eat, drink, drug, sleep to excess, or play video games for hours to try to fill the void. What do you want? Doing something meaningful improves your chances of recovery. Fleeing through substance abuse torpedoes your chances. This chapter covers:

- Value of work or other productive activity.

- Volunteering: benefits and places.
- Return to work (RTW): likelihood, time frame, occupations.
- Success factors for return to productivity.
- Supported employment/other back-to-work programs.
- Government programs to help: SSDI, SSI/PASS, Section 8.
- Retraining/education.
- Electronic brains for job success.
- Getting fired/not hired: reasons and solutions.
- Self-employment: "If no one will hire you, hire yourself."
- Handling rejection.

Value of Work or Other Productive Activity

If you think about what brings you happiness, isn't it more about being productive with your time than loving to work? What is productive activity? Studies define it as all varieties of paid work — full-time, part-time, supported,

> Far and away the best prize that life offers is the chance to work hard at work worth doing.
> — Theodore Roosevelt

sheltered, and self-employment — as well as volunteer work, school, training, and homemaking (Levack et al., 2004).

Not only are you useful if you work, but you're also able to rebuild your social life. What happens if you're not productive? You face the same problems as any unemployed person (Oddy et al., 1985):

- No time structure or network of friends.
- No goals to attain or opportunities to show competence.
- No source of identity or status.

"Okay, fine. I'll work — but where, and doing what?"

Volunteering

Do you want an opportunity to do what you want, where you want, when you want, at a place that wants you? Does this sound impossible and too good to be true? It can happen — just volunteer!

> Service to others is the rent you pay for your life here on earth.
> — Muhammad Ali

Nearly every organization you could imagine actively recruits volunteer workers. Most businesses are less concerned with appearance than performance and prefer substance over style. And most volunteer settings are ideal places to practice vital social and work skills — yes!

Consider this job ad:

- **Wanted:** Volunteer
- **Job description:** Write your own!
- **Location:** Your choice.
- **Requirements:** Clean, sober, eager to help.
- **Hours:** Short. Your choice.
- **Working Conditions:** Pleasant.
- **Benefits:** Work experience, joy, satisfaction, potential for salaried position. Some positions may also include free admission to events!

Benefits of Volunteer Work

Both employers and survivors win on many fronts. Employers win because they always seek good workers, and if they don't need to be paid, it's even better! Perhaps survivors win even more.

"Right, lady. I don't get paid. So, how do I win?"

Volunteer work sites offer perfect opportunities for the socialization practice that we desperately need after our injuries. *You know that your ability to get along and your head took a hit at the same time, don't you?* We can practice our social skills in places that are usually forgiving and friendly. When we're productive, it improves our self-esteem. How? Volunteer work gives us ways to be the helper rather than the helpee — what a concept!

One great example is working with senior citizens who tend to accept, understand, and appreciate a wide range of people. Both as work partners and customers, seniors often welcome opportunities to take on grandparent or helper roles, regardless of who's really the helper. Good listeners — with or without hearing impairments, seniors also enjoy sharing their own war stories. Interactions can be mutually supportive — definitely a win-win situation! And, as retirees, their vocational role is similar to ours — they, too, often seek ways to be of use to others.

Personal experience. Seniors have been very important to my recovery. One I fondly remember is Lucille Carolyn Dare. When I rode my bicycle to church, Lucille always remembered to pick up an afghan for me, so I'd avoid a chill. When Lucille entered a nursing home, it was my turn to help her, and I visited twice a week. Identifying myself as her niece, I had the power of family, so I could directly influence her care. If she needed padding to avoid slumping in her wheelchair or anything else, I spoke with staff members, who usually did as I asked. If nothing changed from one visit to the next, I talked with the supervisor — that worked!! (Surprise, survivors! Our forceful delivery can be very useful!)

Places to Volunteer

Whatever you want to do is wanted somewhere by someone — usually many somewheres and someones! Most organizations continually look for volunteers, gladly accept whatever skills and abilities

> There are no menial jobs, only menial attitudes.
> — William J. Bennett

people offer, and don't ask embarrassing questions. A recent on-line search for "volunteer work" yielded thousands of jobs, including virtual volunteering!

You can organize your search by work site or by work preference. For work site, the "A to Z" choices include: animal shelters, art galleries, churches, clinics, community service centers, day care centers, food banks, homeless shelters, hospices, hospitals, libraries, Meals-On-Wheels, nursing homes, recreation centers, schools, sports teams, symphonies, telephone hot-lines, theaters, and zoos.

If you search by work preference (what you want to do), jobs could include:
- Animals: groom, exercise, rescue, raise puppies.
- Artistic: design, set up, and break down performance stage and props.
- Clerical: answer phones, file, do computer data entry.
- Construction: build, paint, or install various items.
- Environment: plant trees, maintain trails and grounds.
- Maintenance/miscellaneous: clean and repair things, run errands.

- Public relations: greet, sell, assist with presentations, guide, escort, provide respite care, serve as a companion, answer phone hotline, patrol, teach, tutor, mentor, deliver meals.

For those of you who are not able to commit to a schedule, there's still room for you! Many organizations need help for special events — holiday food banks, races, fund drives, etc. Just about any job imaginable is needed, including leadership. Read on!

Personal experience. I love to volunteer! In addition to wearing various church hats (greeter, usher, lay reader, teacher, and choir singer), I've worked with several other organizations, often ushering for performing-arts events. I've even "gonged" the symphony at intermission! Volunteering works for the organizations and for me: I love to be seen as equal to others and not disabled! It's another win-win situation!

Delivery for Meals-On-Wheels was especially enjoyable. We nurtured both body and soul — theirs and our own — and for some of the homebodies, we provided their only social contact for that day.

Another valuable job was responding to calls to a rape hot line about four years after I was sexually assaulted. That I lived through it added to my credibility. I remember reassuring one caller that she wasn't nuts because she needed to sleep with the lights on. Because I'd been there, she believed me when I predicted she'd gradually be able to decrease the amount of light — as I had been able to do. Brain-injury hot lines provide similar opportunities for us to help others walk where we've trod.

Summary of advantages of volunteer work:
- Work is our choice.
- Work is needed.
- Hours are short.
- Demands are few and directions are easy to follow.
- Staff are appreciative.
- Other volunteers are often senior citizens.
- Results are easily achievable and readily noticeable.

- People don't usually get fired! — And being reassigned is not as negative!

Return to Work or Productive Activity

"Okay, lady. I'm convinced I need to work. But I don't want to volunteer. I want to make money! What are my chances? How do I return to work? What can I do?"

You may have heard that the odds of returning to work after brain injury are poor. You can believe this and give up — or ask some questions! Consider these factors in the research that follows:

- Injury factors that affect your chances of return to work.
- Studies measuring likelihood of return to work.
- Time frame for likely return to work.
- Occupations where you are likely to return to work.
- External and internal success factors.

Injury Factors that Affect Your Chances of Return

Severity of injury. Generally, the worse your injury, the less chance of your return to work. But this doesn't mean no chance! For example, a study of 366 survivors found that 38% severe, 66% moderate, and 80% with mild injuries returned to work within two years (Fraser & Wehman, 2001). And, those survivors of severe injury who participate in rehabilitation and/or supported employment programs achieved an employment rate of 50-67%, whether measured short- or long-term (Hoofien et al., 2001; Murrey & Starzinski, 2004; Wehman et al., 1993).

Types and degrees of impairments. Naturally, the kinds and severity of your deficits also impacts your return. Whether you go back to a previous job depends upon what you did, and if you and your employer can agree to modify tasks, hours, and salary.

Studies Measuring Likelihood

When you review research, always ask: who was included, what was their time post-injury, and did they receive support? Where did the study take place and how many participated? What was the definition of "work"? We'll look at exceptionally high (96%), low (25%), and more typical chances of return to productive activity (RTPA) research results.

If you're in the armed forces, you're in good hands. The military was the employer of those in the study with the enviable 96% back-to-work results. These 67 survivors of moderate-to-severe injuries were randomly selected to participate in an eight-week inpatient rehabilitation program with a neuropsychological focus and both individual and group therapy. At one-year follow-up, 96% of program participants had returned to work. Return to duty, where requirements are more stringent, was achieved by 66% (Braverman et al., 1999). These survivors probably experienced some combination of the military taking care of its own, the directive "You will return to work!", and their own drive. Although it would be great if other organizations could duplicate the success, the 96% figure may be atypical, especially for moderate-to-severe survivors.

The low figure reported (25%) by a Singapore study may also be atypical. Though 76% of the 80 participants were severely injured, the study was conducted only one year post-injury — inadequate recovery time to enable return to work (Chua & Kong, 1999). And, in a culture where public gum chewing is disallowed, job accommodations were unlikely!

Contrasting these reports of very low and very high rates of return to work were two studies that found 72% and 78% RTPA. The 72% was achieved by 105 survivors at one year post-injury, 64% with mild-to-moderate injuries. Community integration was important in achieving RTPA for these survivors (Wagner et al., 2002).

A community-based survey found a RTPA of 78% for 107 survivors of 71% severe, 18% moderate, and 11% mild injuries. Respondents either used services or received disability-related publications in San Diego County, California. Injuries occurred 10 or more years previously for 29% of them, with an average time since injury of 7.1 years and a range of one to 30 years. Half of the respondents were over 35 years of age at the time of the interview, with an average age of 38.5 years (Dolen, 1991).

See *Brain Injury Rewiring for Loved Ones* Chapter 12 for a summary of several other studies that predict rate of return to work.

What kinds of productive activities occupied these survivors?
In the Dolen study, of the 78% who were actively working, 18.6% worked for pay (5.6% professionally) or attended school full-time, 59% worked (paid or volunteer) or attended school part-time, and some did both! Common to other survivors was the income reported, with 60% earning less than $10,000. Significantly, despite their injury severity, 81% of the respondents needed no help with self-care and 62% needed no help in home skills, while 65% managed on their own in the community. Nearly 75% walked without help, 16% used a brace or cane, and only 8% used any kind of wheelchair. Importantly, 62% exercised at least three times a week for at least 20 minutes. Atypically, more of these survivors were married both pre- (30%) and post-injury (33%) than most studies and 80% completed some college (26% held advanced degrees).

Time Frame for Return to Productive Activity

Survivors may be slow to return to productive activity, but when we do, we're committed! The percentage of survivors who return to work, either full- or part-time, slowly rises over a period of ten or more years after injury (High et al., 1995). If all productive activity is considered, most of us are engaged or looking for work! And, not only do more of us volunteer our services as time from injury increases, but the percentage of us who attend school or training and work rises as well.

In which occupations do survivors usually work?
Even though we return to work, little is known about what kinds of work we do. Consistent with our need for structure, many survivors of severe injury are employed in the fields of technology and administration. (Hoofien et al., 2001). Some survivors return to professional positions while others work in the trades (Dolen, 1991). Most of those in supported employment positions can be found in warehouse, clerical, and service-related jobs (Wehman et al., 1993). See the Resources in *Brain Injury Rewiring for Loved Ones* Chapter 12.

> The more severe the pain or illness, the more severe will be the necessary changes. These may involve breaking bad habits or acquiring some new or better ones.
> — Peter McWilliams

Success Factors

There are both external and internal factors that will aid or hinder your return to work.

Environmental Factors

As with everything else in our recovery, a successful return to productive activity is a team effort! Important factors (West, 2001) include:

- Returning to the same job and/or employer.
- Flexible work scheduling.
- Environmental modifications.
- Health insurance (after Medicare stops).
- A socially inclusive atmosphere.

Do you notice that you can no longer block out noise when you want to listen to someone or concentrate on a task? *Right! — Me, too!* This is why environmental modifications are important. Post-injury, most of us need to control external disturbances. When audio and/or visual distractions are reduced or eliminated, our brains work better and we're more competent. To help us succeed, it's also important for employers to know that we need to focus on one thing at a time and to work at our own pace (Montgomery, 1995).

Personal experience. Uncontrolled and disturbing environmental stimuli can lead to overload, brain malfunction, and termination. Avoid them! At first I was thrilled to be hired for a full-time position teaching students in an alternative setting — until I saw my "classroom!" It was a former storage room in which the only ventilation and natural light were provided by keeping the door ajar with a wedge — and the steel door stuck in the afternoon heat! Unconnected phone and fax lines hung from the ceiling, tables filled the windowless room, and cupboards and shelves overflowed with folders, papers, outdated textbooks, books, and junk. Several fluorescent lights were burned out, others blinked, and once "school" began, the phone rang frequently — always, it seemed, during instruction. My brain was fried. Unfortunately, my requests to improve this disaster area were considered unessential and a poor use of my preparation time. Without addressing my "request for accommodations,"

I was first placed on administrative leave and then, after five months, given the ultimatum of returning to the same mess. Citing the Americans with Disabilities Act (ADA), I refused.

Internal Success Factors

While environmental factors are largely under the control of others, there are things that we survivors can do to affect our job success. Working with energy and stamina is under our control; these will

> The sun shines not on us, but in us.
> — John Muir

improve with a healthier lifestyle. This means we need to eat nutritious food, be physically active, take snack and stretch breaks, and get the sleep we need. It's no secret that regardless of the setting, we're inconsistent between tasks, days, and even hours of a day. So, do what you can to be at your best!

And, if we want to return to productive activity, we need to get along with others (Prigatano, 1987). You may say, "Not a problem. I can get along with anybody!" Well, that was before your injury. Now some behaviors probably get in the way. We need:

- A capacity for acceptance.
- Self-awareness.
- An ability to regulate emotions.
- Functional independence.

Acceptance of disability is the single most important internal factor in predicting your return to work. It doesn't require employment — it requires an active lifestyle. Not related to time post-injury, acceptance is a continual process of ebb and flow. Immediately after injury, we may think we accept, but it doesn't last. Ever so gradually, we realize that this is reality and deal with it badly or well. We may succumb to depression, substance abuse, and other unhealthy behaviors

> Life is a one-way street. No matter how many detours you take, none of them leads back. And once you know and accept that, life becomes much simpler. Because then you know you must do the best you can with what you have and what you are and what you have become.
> — Isabel Moore

during this process. The lucky ones among us connect with others who value us for who we are and not for what we do. We often feel that because we are not who we were that we are less as human brings. Not true!

My brother and sister survivors, hear this — each person has an intrinsic, God-given goodness! And despite injury-caused impairments in various functions, this essence and wholeness cannot be destroyed by any amount of damage to the body and mind. When we seek to understand the reason for the injury, we often blame God or ourselves — or both — and believe that our essence has been damaged. Not!

Personal experience. *In the Emotional Rewiring chapter, I recollected an "aha" moment that changed my thinking, self-image, and behavior. I was selected by God — not picked on — because I'm strong.*

Self-awareness is the second best internal predictor of employability. It takes courage to confront the reality of how our brain injuries changed us. But we must move past denial to acceptance to rejoin society.

The ability to regulate your emotions and functional independence are also significant internal success factors for working again (Nat'l Inst. Disability & Rehab. Research, 1994). No need to explain why we can't still expect to be employed or make friends after we explode, right?

Someone who is functionally independent displays the abilities to wash, dress, groom, toilet, and feed himself. He is also able to arrange transportation to arrive places on time, with little or no supervision. How does someone achieve functional independence? Persevere. Participate in real-life activities such as meal preparation and clean-up. Stay determined to rewire and be patient — with yourself and others. Remember the prediction about better days will come — if we don't quit.

To summarize: you are ready for employment when you demonstrate:

- Capacity for acceptance.
- Self-awareness.
- Self-control.
- Functional independence.

SAFER — Stop, Assess, Fix, Evaluate, Retry

"Okay, fine. I know about the essential work qualities. How do I know if I possess them?" The same SAFER method we used to rewire our cognitive, emotional, and social selves applies to the vocational and community re-entry area. In fact, successfully returning to productive activity demands its use! Let's apply it to work.

Stop: First, we stop our actions — physical, mental, and emotional.

Assess: Then with the help of others, we analyze our situation:
- If we don't like where we are or if we're stuck in limbo, we ask where we want to go and how we get there.
- Positive factors — what is working — and possible reasons.
- Negative factors — what isn't working — and possible reasons.
- Potential changes in us and/or the environment.

Next, we prioritize our change list. For example, if we seek a specific job, we need to know the requirements and if we meet them or can achieve them with additional training.

Fix: We change/request help in one or more of the unworkable parts:
- Internal immediate: grooming, energy level, physical health.
- Internal dynamic: emotional awareness and control, social skills, work habits and abilities.
- External environment: hours, ambiance (space/light), distractions (visual/auditory), duties, requirements/demands (speed/complexity).

Evaluate: We examine the changes we've made. If they work, we keep them and keep going. If not, we discard them.

Retry: Based on our evaluation, we try new interventions and repeat the process, if necessary.

Personal experience. When I recently lamented to friends that I approached writing this chapter with trepidation, the response was, "Why? You're an expert at 'Job Search.' It's the 'Job Find' that you have trouble with!" This comment is both funny and true. After more than 30 years of searching for "the right job," I'm still knocking on doors.

The doors and their locks have changed in size, color, combination, and number. Some have even opened for a short time — the average time is about six weeks. But I'm still tripping over the threshold or missing — or choosing to miss — the first turn in the corridor. "The right one" hasn't stayed opened yet — or, at least, I haven't seen it.

So, what's my plan? Follow SAFER, look for other doors to open, and seek combinations that I haven't tried recently. The journey seems endless, but — as I've said many times before — at least I'm still on it.

Work and Vocational Service Programs

Supported Employment

If you want to return to work, this is the most effective way to do it (Wehman et al., 2003). Participation in work programs where staff are specially trained and the jobs are appropriate results in 50-70% of the survivors reentering the competitive work force (West, 1995). Wow!

Not only do we reenter the work force, but we stay employed! One study over a 14-year time period reported that 59 survivors with moderate to severe injuries averaged 42.58 months of employment. These workers earned more than $26,000 on average, over this time-period, which averaged to $17,000 more than the costs of the program! (Wehman et al., 2003). Another group with severe injuries worked 75% of the total available months in competitive employment after involvement in supported employment services with an on-site specialist. Job retention was 71% for this group of 41 survivors! (Nat'l Inst. Disability Research Office, 1994).

"Whoa, this sounds great! Maybe I can actually work in a job I like and be paid for it! Tell me more."

What is supported employment? What are the job requirements?
Supported employment means working for pay while receiving support services such as job coaching, transportation, individual supervision, and assistive technology. Importantly, to help us maintain employment,

support is never completely removed — it is decreased as warranted by job performance, and as we gain skills and confidence.

Job coaches provide specialized, on-site training to teach workers how to perform the job and adjust to the environment. On-site training includes job skills and work-related behaviors, including social skills.

At least 18 hours per week must be worked to participate and to earn the same benefits as other paid employees, like sick leave, vacation time, health benefits, and bonuses. To locate a program, contact your local Vocational Rehabilitation agency (US Dept of Labor, 2005).

Social Security Ticket-to-Work Program

This is a flexible and voluntary federal vocational service program for those who receive either SSDI or SSI disability benefits. *See important information about SSDI and SSI in the next section.* If you participate in the program and meet certain requirements, benefits continue and no medical disability reviews occur. However, benefits can be terminated if your annual earnings exceed what is called Substantial Gainful Activity (SGA), which was $970 in 2009 (Social Security, 2008). Contact Social Security if you want a "ticket"!

State Vocational Rehabilitation Agency

Your state agency can provide various services, including vocational testing, counseling, and financial help toward education or training as a member of the Employment Network in the Ticket-to-Work Program. Program rules change, so maintain contact with your counselor.

Personal experience. Vocational Rehabilitation provided me with guidance, counseling, and money for school. My first counselor, Cathy Wallace, truly had my best interests at heart and wasn't either intimidated by my mouth or blown away by my frustrated outbursts. Keep looking for people with whom you feel comfortable — they can be found!

Governmental Programs

Social Security — SSDI and SSI

Disability benefits can be the key to your economic survival — be glad we have them in the USA! As soon as possible after the injury, contact the Social Security Administration (SSA). You can call 1-800-772-1213 or apply through the Social Security website (www.ssa.gov/disability). Determine your eligibility for all Social Security programs by completing the BEST screening tool on the website.

Two federal programs pay disability benefits: Social Security Disability Income (SSDI) and Supplemental Security Income (SSI). To qualify for SSDI, you are at least 22 years old and paid into the FICA system when you worked (if wages qualified). If you were disabled before age 22, you qualify if your parent(s) paid into the system or your parent(s) receive either disability or retirement benefits or is deceased. To qualify for SSI, your income and resources must be limited.

Personal experience. Amazingly enough, I recall no one — until I moved to California — telling me about Social Security for years after my injury, even though I lived in both Minnesota and Texas after the injury, used (or attempted to use) various state agencies, and had contributed to the system through various teaching jobs before the injury. Despite a 1976 injury, I didn't receive benefits until 1987.

Don't let this happen to you! Benefits are available only after you are officially considered "disabled," regardless of what you think is fair. If you are denied benefits, appeal. If you disagree with the decision by the first official, you still retain the right to a hearing with an Administrative Law Judge. There is also a Decision Review Board to review and correct decisional errors (Social Security Online, 2006).

Why reapply? Most applicants (about 2/3) are denied benefits the first time. Many of us didn't know this ugly little fact and waited years to reapply. Also, about 90% of all first appeals are denied. But about 70% of those who persevere ultimately receive their benefits (Abrams, 1999). Keep trying and do not give up!

Do I need to hire an attorney? What is the cost?
Do you want to win your appeal? If you are denied benefits, contact an attorney as soon as possible. You improve your chances of winning if you are represented. The attorney prepares the case and prepares you to testify convincingly — critical for those of us who don't look disabled. Legal fees are usually 25% of past-due benefits. If the case is lost, no fee is paid, except out-of-pocket copying, etc.

> *Personal experience. Thanks to my attorney, I finally received SSDI benefits — 12 years after my injury. It took that long mostly because of two factors: ignorance — mine and others' — of how the system works and the fact that head injury wasn't considered a disability then.*

Supplemental Security Income (SSI)
You qualify for this cash assistance program if you have few resources, are blind, disabled, or age 65 or older. Nationwide, the monthly cash assistance rates for 2009 are $674 for an individual and from $1011 for a couple, with yearly increases. The amount of your benefit depends upon where you live; some states supplement the basic amount.

Resources, not including auto or home and attached land must not exceed $2000 for single people or $3000 for couples. Any retirement accounts must be exhausted before you can be eligible.

To determine benefit amount, money not counted includes the first $20 of most income received in a month, the first $65 earned from employment and half the amount over $65, home energy assistance, food stamps, and the cost of food and clothing from non-profit organizations.

Employment affects both SSDI and SSI benefits in several ways. It's complicated. See *Brain Injury Rewiring for Loved Ones* for more details. If you want to go to school or obtain training, SSI can help in two ways.

The SSI student earned-income exclusion.
This is good news for students! If you are under age 22 and regularly attend school, you can earn $640 in one month in 2009 (an increase of 5.8% from 2008) or $6600 in 2009 without affecting either eligibility or benefits. "Regularly attend" means you attend at least eight hours a week in college or at least 12 hours a week in a training course to prepare you

for employment. You also may qualify if you are homebound due to disability (Social Security Online).

The SSI Plan to Achieve Self-Support (PASS).
This is a terrific program where you can "set aside" income or resources for a specified period of time so you can pursue a work goal. For example: you could set aside money to pay expenses for education, vocational training, or to start a business, as long as the expenses are related to achieving your work goal.

Under your PASS, the income that you set aside is not counted in determining your SSI payment amount. And, the resources that you set aside aren't counted when they determine your initial and continuing eligibility for SSI either.

Another benefit is that a PASS can help you establish or maintain SSI eligibility and can increase your SSI payment amount. For example: if you receive $800 in SSDI, you have too much income for SSI. But if you otherwise qualify for SSI and have a work goal, you could use some of your SSDI to pay for PASS expenses. That could reduce your income enough to be eligible for SSI! The result will be a higher monthly cash benefit with eligibility for both SSDI and SSI. (PASS money won't increase your SSI benefit if you already receive the full benefit amount). Use form SSA-545-BK to apply (Social Security Online, 2008).

You can apply for PASS if you receive SSI or could qualify for it. If you're eligible for SSI and have income or resources other than what's needed for living expenses, you qualify. You may not need a PASS now, but you may need one in the future to remain eligible or to increase your SSI payment amount.

The PASS can include transportation, attendant care, childcare, education or training, vocational services, adaptive equipment (including computer), tutor, job coach, uniforms, medical expenses, or supplies to start a business. It is designed to help people acquire those items, services, or skills to compete with able-bodied people for an entry-level job in a professional, business, or trade environment. The goal job must produce sufficient earnings to reduce dependency on SSI payments. A helpful pamphlet entitled *Working While Disabled — A Plan for*

Achieving Self-Support (SSA Publication No. 05-11017) is available online at www.ssa.gov/pubs/11017.html.

PASS requirements. (Social Security Online, 2008) You must:
- Be eligible for SSI (low or no income).
- Have another source of income besides SSI that can be excluded: wages or Social Security Disability.

The PASS must:
- Be in writing and approved by Social Security, which prefers that you use their form, the SSA-545-BK. You can get copies of the PASS form at your local office, or from the Social Security website (www.ssa.gov).
- Be reviewed by Social Security periodically to assure that your plan is actually helping you progress toward self-support.
- Include a specific work goal that you are capable of performing.
- Include a specific time frame for reaching your goal.
- Show what money (besides SSI payments) and other resources you have or receive that you will use to reach your goal.
- Show how your money and resources will be used.

The PASS funds:
- Must be separate from other funds, i.e. in a separate account.
- Must be spent only on approved items listed in the PASS.
- Must be recorded in an organized manner.
- Must be documented with receipts.
- Can be used for installment payments or down payment for a vehicle, wheelchair, or computer.
- Will not count against your resource limit ($2000 individual).
- Are not counted in determining SSI benefit amount.

My recommendations for PASS success:
- Prove that goal is achievable with reference letters from professionals (teachers, counselors, doctors, clergy).
- Show interest and ability (transcripts, work samples, resume).
- Document anticipated expenses with written statements from reputable sources (computer store, trade dealer).

- Practice your presentation with others.
- Ask a respected professional/friend to accompany you to your PASS meeting with the SSI representative.
- If the first PASS is denied, appeal with more documentation or submit a new plan.

Personal experience. This incentive really helped me! Fortunately, my Vocational Rehabilitation counselor, Cathy Wallace, referred me to her friend, Terry Knorr, a knowledgeable counselor in the ACCESS San Diego office, who wrote my first PASS. Charming and experienced, Terry was able to convince the SSI worker to work with a brain-injury survivor. Acceptance of my PASS took two tries, but with Terry's help, we succeeded. My PASS plan enabled me to purchase a computer, printer, and assorted office furniture as well as pay school expenses. Thanks to the experience gained from working with Terry, I wrote my own second PASS, which paid for schooling and books. PASS works!

Subsidized Housing through HUD Section 8

If your income is reduced — whether or not you qualify for SSI — immediately apply for the federal subsidized housing program called Section 8. This program makes up the difference between what we can afford to pay (usually considered 30% of our income) and the current rental rates. The usual waiting list is 5 years, so apply now!

Personal experience. I've been a grateful recipient of Section 8 housing assistance for over 15 years. Housing workers patiently adjust my rental portion to reflect changing medical expenses and my numerous attempts to support myself with various jobs. I always feel heard.

However, when searching for a rental with a Section 8 housing voucher, I've felt unwanted many times. After hearing, "Oh no, we don't accept that!" — it takes a lot of positive self-talk to feel OK and sometimes many months to find someone willing to rent to me. Keep trying!

Retraining/education

Most survivors who successfully return to work — even for a short time — obtain some type of retraining or education.

> Let me tell you the secret that has led me to my goal. My strength lies in my tenacity.
> — Louis Pasteur

Whether you want to return to your original area of work or others that are similar — but less demanding — improving your skills increases your marketability. For example, a degreed professional may earn an assistant certificate at a community college to continue in the same work, but at a lower level of responsibility.

Attend school after injury. How?

"Return to school with a memory deficit? Pulleeeez! I can't even find the place, let alone learn there! I'll need a lot of help to be able to perform." What shall I do?

- Meet with the counselors at the disabled students' service center.
- Inform your instructors about your brain injury.

To improve the likelihood that they'll help, contact them before class starts. Most educators appreciate any information that helps them succeed in their job, which is teaching students. So, by helping ourselves, we also help them — a win-win situation! And when we tell instructors of our needs, it alerts them to the possibility that other students may need accommodations, too.

What is the most effective way to inform them? Bring relevant written materials from your local brain-injury association. Keep your goal in mind. This is not a "here's my story" opportunity, although you may be asked. Your goal is to inform, request extra exam time, and whatever else you may need. Hopefully, some of the psychological tests you took profiled these educational needs. Consider your instructor's needs (time and material overload).

Personal experience. I was fortunate that the director of the rehab clinic at SDSU was brain-injury savvy. He informed a wary professor about my strengths and weaknesses, thus paving the way for dialogue and enabling us both to be successful. Following his intercession, Prof. Wary turned into Prof. Helpful.

Attend school after injury. What kind?

Any training that improves your skills, whether short-term, long-term, technical, or degree-oriented, will help prepare you for successful vocational re-entry. It's your choice!

If returning to your original field of work is not realistic or you don't want to work at a lower level, part-time, or on-call, there are more options! Look at interests — past or current — to seek another area to pursue. If you love cars, for example, part-time auto mechanics programs are offered at community colleges. The computer field also offers many different areas to pursue. Do you love to teach or care for others? Many opportunities in education and nursing-related fields await you!

Personal experience. Immediately after my injury in Minnesota, I enrolled in our local community colleges to take classes in study skills and reading improvement, in addition to karate and river floating, in my continued search for balance — and fun!

When I arrived in San Diego, it was only natural to continue my health/fitness career path, since the social work field offered fewer opportunities than in the past. First, I pursued a massage technician's license and began course work in Corporate Fitness. Then I took courses for a recognized fitness certificate, which I needed to work as a trainer, despite undergraduate work in physical education. Following success in these challenging programs, I felt confident enough to enroll in a Master's degree program in a growing field with available jobs (special education). With hard work, I completed the program in less than a year!

Personal experience. My partial post-injury job history: Many people, particularly my parents (who paid for my college education and teaching credential), misunderstood my repeated attempts to find and keep work. During a ten-year period, the jobs I remember included: direct (door-to-door) sales of cable TV and children's reading programs, cocktail waitress (many times), bookkeeper, cashier, phone book deliverer, attendant for bed-ridden people, sales of bicycles and fitness equipment, phone sales of smoking-cessation programs, door-to-door social researcher, grocery-store coupon distributor, trolley ticket system demonstrator, HUD interviewer (of clients in dangerous urban areas), co-therapist with phobic clients (one with inability to urinate in a public restroom), auto and truck detailer, psychotherapist, ghostwriter/editor on spec (may or may not get paid).

What aren't included in this past job list are numerous moneymaking opportunities that involved the medical community such as selling my plasma, submitting to various biopsies, or participating in 12-hour blood reinfusion studies. Such cash opportunities varied from $5 per donation for plasma to $100 for biopsies to $200 for two all-day blood reinfusion studies. (When asked why I allowed a biopsy to be taken, my only reply was "For $100.")

I no doubt earned some sort of "survivor-perseverance medal" for donating plasma five times in a month in 1980 to earn an extra $5, which went towards the purchase of new running shoes.

Not all survivors are this determined or crazy or stupid — pick a word! — but we all feel we are.

While variations in pre-injury personality, abilities, and socio-economic status are as great as the age span of survivors, one overwhelming constant is this feeling of not being OK, or, as quoted earlier: "I knew something was terribly wrong, and I was that something!" Continual reminders of our internal goodness may be needed for a long time.

Electronic Brains for Job Success

"Oh sure! Return to work with my brain? I don't think so! I have trouble remembering the day of the week, let alone how to do my job! I'll need a lot of help to be able to perform."

Who said brains need be human? Electronic brains to the rescue! How about a computer program? The expert shell system, used for years by government and business, provides a structure for work tasks:

- Tasks that require decision-making are formulated into a set of rules.
- Rules are inputted into the shell program.
- This program develops a rule structure to implement the decisions.

What are the drawbacks to these computer programs?

- You are dependent upon the computer and software to function.
- You are very specifically trained.
- Work tasks must be reduced to a set of rules with few exceptions.
- Your employer must approve use of the device to perform the job.
- You must become capable of doing your job using the program.

Getting Fired/Not Hired

Can you relate to these words? It's difficult to describe what it feels like to be fired 13 times — in one year! Even if the jobs were inappropriate, getting fired feels more or less the same every time — awful. After all, who likes rejection, even if the job was a poor fit?

> I just wish they'd tell me I'm running out of straws before it's the last one!
> — Author

Fired

Wrong job, wrong time, wrong place, and — wrong personality.
Although the reasons for my firings varied, my post-injury personality usually played a part. Some causes included: being too honest, working too hard, not getting along, inexperience, not fitting in, working too hard, telling off the wrong people, seeking excellence, not getting along, working too hard — get the idea?

With some of the firings, I still don't have a clue about the reason and each rejection eroded my self-confidence a little more.

Self-talk. What we say to ourselves is often far worse than what anyone says to us, especially after just getting fired. For example, "I'm not good enough to even do...", "I can't even keep a lousy job doing...", "Why did I do (or say) that?"

Personal experience. My beloved, former principal, Don Sonsalla, hired me after my injury because I had worked with him before it. When he told me that if I spoke the same way to the kids that I spoke to myself I wouldn't be a

> Let me listen to me and not to them.
> — Gertrude Stein

good teacher or keep my job, it made me think about what I said to myself. I changed to positive self-talk, and am now a lot easier going and much happier.

We can also view getting fired/not hired as we do former friends who drop us before we drop them: "they did me a favor because I didn't like the job anyway!" If someone doesn't want us, sooner or later we probably won't want them either.

Not Getting Hired

Knowing why we're not hired is important to learn. One special education supervisor kindly told me years after our first interview that she remembered "you just didn't seem quite right. Your social skills have really improved since that time. You seemed to try too hard."

She was exactly right — isn't that sad? "You tried too hard!" We all try so hard — we desperately want to fit in, to get along like we used to. This is another area where we need to realize our loss, grieve it, and keep working to gain the skills we need so we can be more relaxed.

After the candid appraisal, this department head requested me as a substitute teacher. I loved working with her because she liked me, my work ethic, and she included me in lunch and party plans!

Not knowing why is worse because we don't know what we need to do to get hired! Did I do too much or try too hard? Was I too thorough or too honest? Did I lack tact when talking to someone? Did I not follow the rules, spoken or unspoken? Did I forget to focus on my job and talk instead about my life and/or injury?

SAFER: Work with loved ones and therapists/counselors to analyze both getting fired and not hired. — You could list this exploration as a goal for work reentry with your Vocational Rehabilitation counselor! Honestly share your ideas so that they can help support your growth and acquisition of needed skills. The SAFER plan will help you stay positive as you determine what needs to be "fixed" so you can retry!

Self-Employment

Is one of your SAFER career-fix ideas to be your own boss? For some of us, this is a good idea! If we view not getting hired and getting fired as a gift, we can reframe those negatives experiences into a positive: "Maybe this is just the push I need to employ myself!"

> If no one will hire you, hire yourself.
> — Steve Wilders

To make our venture successful, we first need to develop a plan. Ask your Vocational Rehab counselor about the agencies that provide free technical assistance. Not only can self-employment be listed as a work goal for a PASS, but financial aid may be available from other places!

Advantages. Many positive aspects of self-employment that are helpful for non-disabled people are necessary for survivors. Some of these include: flexible schedule, hospitable environment, no need for travel, an ability to take exercise or nap breaks, and — perhaps most importantly — the opportunity to work the hours our biorhythms prefer — start late or work in the evening. An added bonus is only dealing with those people we choose, rather than enduring the stress of unaccepting co-workers or bosses.

Disadvantages. The usual problems for self-employed people are magnified for us, not the least of which is very limited financial capital, unless you received a large injury settlement. Perhaps generous family members and friends can also help you. Our tendency to be trusting and rather grandiose can also lead to problems, as can our typical memory and organizational (executive function) difficulties.

Caveats. Be honest in your self-appraisal of whether self-employment is realistic for you. (*I know I tend to be easily ripped off, buy in quantity — if one is good, 10 seem to be better! — and I make foolish decisions regarding my limited resources.*) If you do embrace the idea of self-employment, be sure to surround yourself with others who can help you with the business aspects and/or develop the skills you need to be successful. Perhaps partnering with or hiring someone to do the bookkeeping can be part of your plan, if this is difficult for you.

Personal experience. A while ago I literally ran into a real go-getter, a Senior Director for Mary Kay Cosmetics, at a flute concert at my church. After this divine intervention I, too, began to sell Mary Kay skincare and cosmetics as an independent contractor. Thanks to a generous loan from my adopted sister, Marlys, I could purchase organizing cases and inventory to start me on my way. This works for me because selling is a lifelong skill, my own skincare products are half-price, I make a little money, and it's fun!

Handling Rejection

No longer do I place the importance that I used to on steady employment or having a real job — I decided that if it's the right job, it'll be mine, and if not, it won't. So far, the right real job hasn't jumped out at

> No one can make you feel inferior without your consent.
> — Eleanor Roosevelt

me. Shall I reevaluate my career plan? I'm still knocking on those doors. It's just that now I'm not trying to knock them down! Remember that if the door locks baffle you, one of your friends can usually interpret.

If you feel constantly rejected by employers, keep doing what energizes and relaxes you, remediate your social skills, and remember the positive self-talk. Just do it! You can rewire!

Personal experience. A few years ago I asked myself "Am I where I want to be or thought I would be after 25 years?" The answer was "No." But thanks to my former therapist, Christine Baser, PhD, I could also ask, "Am I okay with where I am?" Yes! "Do I even sort of accept where I am?" Yes, because I did my best and so did all the people on my lifeline. "Am I resigned to remaining here?" No. Never will I stop trying.

I can answer this question more positively today because I've (mostly) enjoyed writing Brain Injury Rewiring and I (mostly) like my one-day-a-week work as a personal fitness trainer. I'm still guiding the same stroke survivor after nearly 3 years! I followed my heart — and didn't give up on myself. With a little bit of luck, the following qualities will to lead a productive life for you, too.

Summary

To succeed, you need:
* Self-awareness.

- Self-acceptance.
- Self-control.
- Continuous training.
- Perseverance.
- Assistance from God and others.

Checklist of requirements to rewire vocationally:

- Be productive to improve your quality of life.
- Volunteer to be the helper rather than the helpee.
- Accepting your disability requires an active lifestyle.

> There are no menial jobs, only menial attitudes.
> — William J. Bennett

- Learn to regulate your emotions and be independent.
- Use SAFER to successfully return to productive activity.
- Supported employment helps you return to work.
- Make use of Social Security's Ticket to Work Program.
- Utilize your state's Vocational Rehabilitation agencies.
- Apply for SSDI and SSI, and if you are denied benefits, appeal!
- Apply for a SSI PASS.
- Apply for subsidized housing through HUD Section 8.
- Obtain retraining/education.
- Explore new/different career fields.
- If you're not hired and/or are fired, remember what Eleanor Roosevelt said: "No one can make you feel inferior without your consent."
- Consider self-employment.

You can do it! You can rewire!

Conclusion

Dear brain-injury survivors,

I hope that *Brain Injury Rewiring for Survivors* helped — and will help — you to optimally recover from your brain injury. My intention was to provide a

> Do not let what you cannot do interfere with what you can do.
> — Coach John Wooden

lifeline to new connections for you because rehabilitation will undoubtedly be the most challenging work of your life. Just remember: "Don't underestimate willpower. It can move a mountain or two."

You've learned ways to rewire body, mind, and spirit that will improve your life — if you follow them. Help your loved ones to help you by doing your best!

I ask you to aid other survivors in their recoveries by sharing what you know, encouraging them on their journeys, and continuing to search for more answers. My hope is that everyone has an opportunity to not just survive the climb, but also to breathe the clean mountain air, feel the sunshine, smell the blossoms, and enjoy the scenery along the way. See Resources to find the connections you need. May God bless us on our journeys! To provide a ready reference to the many ideas and strategies in *Brain Injury Rewiring for Survivors*, the most important ones are listed here:

General Rewiring

- Believe in yourself.
- You still possess a few billion neurons ready for a "work order."
- Remember Sir Charles Symonds' words: "It is not the kind of injury that matters, but the kind of head."

> All things are possible until they are proved impossible — and even the impossible may only be so, as of now.
> — Pearl S. Buck

293

- Create a healthy environment with lots of natural light and plants.
- Some improvement can occur even years after an injury.
- Work at getting better.
- "Use it or lose it!" and never ever quit!
- Find out what is and is not possible to change.
- Establish short-term and long-term goals.

Spiritual

- Chart your heart.
- Play the music that's best for each of your activities.
- Learn what sounds and noises overload your wires, then flee, fight, or negotiate.

> When you can't solve the problem, manage it.
> — Rev. Robert H. Schuller

- Pray!
- Find healing practices that work for you — and do them!
- Explore the arts and other expressive activities.

Cognitive

- Use all your senses — say, hear, see, do — to reinforce memory.
- Use positive and encouraging self-talk.

> Happiness is a thing to be practiced, like the violin.
> — John Lubbock

- Keep a calendar and notebook to log important information.
- Do Sudoku and crossword puzzles to stimulate your brain, re-establish logic patterns, improve visual tracking, and for fun!
- Find what your needs are: best time of day (for activities, people, and places), food (how frequently to eat and what kinds of food), activity (amount, frequency, and duration), sleep/rest (amount of sleep/rest periods during the day).
- Spend time alone — share your experiences or not!
- Set up your environment for success.
- Eat healthfully.
- Exercise — mentally and physically — every day.

- Do not veg out in front of the TV.
- Use SAFER (Stop, Assess, Fix, Examine, Retry) to solve problems.
- Know that you can fix your brain — if you work at it.

Emotional

- Avoid known causes of distress.
- Ask, "What do I need to be calm?"
- Ask, "Who can help me?"
- Practice a ritual like meditation, yoga, or tai chi.
- Structure daily activities to feel some control.
- Consider ways to cope before you blow your circuits.
- Find and use verbal support.
- Remember that it's the physical damage that causes you to fail at something, not that you're not trying.
- Recall motivational words from respected sources.
- Listen to motivational audio or video tapes.
- Display visual reminders that express positive messages to provide a lift, like "You're a winner!"
- Considering owning a pet. *Fish are easy!*
- Seek community enrichment resources and use them!
- Get active — do anything that brings you joy!
- Don't use/abuse substances like tobacco, alcohol, drugs.
- Grieving and accepting your loss may take many years.
- Believe that you are okay — just different from what you were.
- Know that you can be better — but only if you work at it.
- Work on recovery by strengthening some abilities, compensating for others, and adapting your environment.

> Often we look so long at the closed door that we don't see the one that has opened for us.
> — Patricia Neal

Conventional and Alternative Medicine

- Keep looking until you find healers you like.
- Be open to different methods, therapies, and devices.

> Absence of proof isn't proof of absence!
> — Nathan Zasler

- Trust your gut when choosing therapies and helpers.
- Be prepared for your appointments.
- Don't act/talk like a victim.
- Practice SAFER.

Nutritional

- To nurture "my body, my car," choose good foods.
- Learn about healthful eating.

> You are what you eat.
> — Adelle Davis

- Develop a nutrition plan.
- Eat slowly. Eat lots of brain food: fish, fruits, and veggies.
- Eat only when hungry.
- Eat several small meals a day.
- Avoid junk food.
- Consume no more than 30% of total calories from fat and 10% from saturated fat, and avoid trans fat, if possible.
- Don't smoke!
- Avoid stimulating activities, people, food, or drink late in the evening.
- Finish vigorous exercise at least three hours before going to bed.
- Maintain regular arising and sleeping hours.
- Keep lights low to prepare body and brain for sleep.
- Enjoy a small snack if hungry.
- Relax with light reading, soft music, or a warm bath.
- Keep bedroom cool, quiet, inviting, and dark.
- To quiet body and mind, use the white noise of a fan and the Chinese medicine technique of touching your fingertips in a teepee shape, while you lie on your side or back.
- If sleepless after 20 minutes or so, get up. Read or make a to-do list for the next day. Making a plan relieves anxious thoughts.
- If you awaken, recite a mantra, breathe deeply, practice relaxation exercises, fantasize, or think other pleasant thoughts.

Physical

- Just do it!
- Find what activities you like — and do one or two daily.
- Schedule activities on your calendar.
- Do relaxation activities like yoga, qigong, or tai chi.
- Use RICE, pressure-point, and self-massage techniques.

> Every day you do one of two things: build health or produce disease in yourself.
> — Adelle Davis

Social

- Know that you can make friends again.
- Socialize in friendly places.
- Practice your social skills in therapy and in real-world places.

> Never let the fear of striking out get in your way!
> — Babe Ruth

- Draw a target to select the best people to socialize with.
- Choose social interactions with a high chance for success.
- Show interest with eye contact, enthusiasm, and posture.
- Be prepared for questions when you date — or otherwise.
- Just because someone asks a question doesn't mean you're required to answer it in any lengthy manner.
- Ask others "why?", "how?", and opinion questions.
- Remember: the best defense is a good offense.
- Observe the behavior of those you admire and ask them for tips.
- Know that our social difficulties lie with what we do rather than what we are.
- Respect, graciousness, and friendliness overcome most social errors.
- Be a receiver, not just a broadcaster!
- Fake it till you make it.
- There's hope to improve sexual dysfunction after injury.
- If you feel overloaded, either internally or externally, leave the situation immediately or ask for help.
- "Behavior change precedes attitude change."
- Prepare your body, mind, and spirit for outings, with sleep, good nutrition, exercise, and readiness.

- Interact with six or more people per day.
- Be active in many pursuits.
- Practice SAFER (Stop, Assess, Fix, Evaluate, Retry).
- We can learn new behaviors — our brains are "plastic."
- Not all social glitches result from our mistakes.
- Open, affirming, and welcoming people and places do exist!
- Keep knocking on doors to find welcoming people and places.

Vocational

- Be productive to improve your quality of life.
- Volunteer to be the helper rather than the helpee.
- Acceptance of disability requires an active lifestyle.
- Learn to regulate your emotions and be functionally independent.
- Apply the SAFER plan to successfully return to productive activity.

> I am only one. But still I am one. I cannot do everything, But still I can do something; And because I cannot do everything, I will not refuse to do something that I can do.
> — Edward Everett Hale

- Consider supported employment to return to work.
- Take advantage of the Social Security Ticket-to-Work Program.
- Use your state's Vocational Rehabilitation agencies.
- Apply for SSDI and SSI, and if you are denied benefits, appeal!
- Apply for a SSI PAS.
- Apply for HUD Section 8 subsidized housing.
- Obtain retraining/education.
- Explore new/different career fields.
- If you're not hired and/or fired, remember what Eleanor Roosevelt said: "No one can make you feel inferior without your consent."
- Consider self-employment

> Success isn't a result of spontaneous combustion. You must set yourself on fire.
> — Arnold H. Glasow

You can do it! You can rewire!

Resources

Organizations that can help with all phases of brain injury rewiring are listed first in this section. Following that, resources are arranged in the same order as the chapters.

Go to www.rewiring.org for up-to-date recovery information and resources that also include books and DVDs.

General and Disability Information

American Association of People with Disabilities (AAPD)
> The largest cross-disability member organization in the US. Offers many benefits.
> www.aapd.com, 800-840-8844

American Brain Tumor Association
> Promotes research and offers information and support.
> www.abta.org, 800-886-2282

American Stroke Association (a division of American Heart Association)
> Information & resources for both survivors and caregivers; free subscription to *Stroke Connection Magazine*. Links include a national network of local support groups.
> www.strokeassociation.org, 888-4-STROKE ((888-478-7653)

Brain Injury Association, USA
> Provides information, education, and support to survivors, loved ones, and professionals. Many state affiliates, local chapters and support groups.
> www.biausa.org, 800-444-6443

Brainline.org
> Information on preventing, treating, and living with traumatic brain injury; funded by the Defense and Veterans Brain Injury Center.
> www.brainline.org, 703-998-2020

Centre for Neuro Skills
> Offers information, resources, services, products, and rehab programs for TBI. Products include: cognitive software, one-handed keyboard, vision restoration therapy device. Its TBI Resource Guide is the largest on-line bookstore for TBI.
> www.neuroskills.com, 800-922-4994

Disability-Related Information and Resources: This federal website provides comprehensive information about programs, services, laws and benefits in nine areas that include education, employment, health, housing, technology, and transportation. Find state and local resources in all these areas using a map.
> www.disabilityinfo.gov, various phone numbers on website.

Disability Resources Monthly (DRM)
> Guide to Disability Resources on the Internet. Updated daily. Provides well-organized access to thousands of resources for independent living arranged by state and subdivided by topic.
> www.disabilityresources.org, contact information on website.

Epilepsy Foundation of America (EFA)
> Provides information, resources, advocacy, and links to local foundations.
> www.efa.org, 800-332-1000

Family Village: A Global Community of Disability-Related Resources
> User-friendly website that integrates information, adaptive products, technology, recreational activities, education.
> www.familyvillage.wisc.edu/

Healthfinder (US Dept. of Health & Human Services)
> General health information on over 1600 topics from trusted sources. Find services and information. Free health interactive tools.
> www.healthfinder.gov/

Lash & Associates Publishing/Training
Traumatic brain injury books, brain injury information, and
resources.
www.lapublishing.com, 919-562-0015

National Health Information Center (NHIC)
A resource database and referral service to link you with
organizations that can answer health questions.
www.health.gov/nhic (various phone numbers on the site)

National Institute of Neurological Disorders and Stroke (NINDS)
Information on disorders from A to Z, materials, research,
resources.
www.ninds.nih.gov, 800-352-9424

National Rehabilitation Information Center (NARIC)
Offers an abundance of resources: employment, advocacy,
benefits, financial assistance, education, technology, and more.
www.naric.com, 800-346-2742

New Horizons Un-Limited
More than 2500 international links to information, products,
resources, guides, events, programs, reference library, news;
includes technology, recreation, arts, education, employment.
www.new-horizons.org

Traumatic Brain Injury National Resource Center (NRCTBI)
Helpful information for survivors and loved ones that includes
personalized responses to questions, articles, products,
conferences, links, FAQs.
www.neuro.pmr.vcu.edu

United Cerebral Palsy (UCP)
Information and resources in many areas, including products and
services; research and advocacy for people with all disabilities.
www.ucp.org, 800-872-5827

United Spinal Association (USA)
Over 1900 sources of information/products on its
usatechguide.org site; offers links, services.
www.unitedspinal.org, 800-404-2898

Family/Loved Ones

Family Caregiver Alliance (FCA)
> National Center on Caregiving. Education, information, services, research, and advocacy for caregivers; state-by-state guide of available help from all sources.
> www.caregiver.org, 800-445-8106

National Family Caregivers Association.
> Educates, supports, empowers, and advocates for all caregivers. Home of statewide Caregiving Community Action Network.
> www.nfcacares.org, 800-896-3650

Southern Caregiver Resource Center (CRC)
> Information, referral, support groups, counseling, consultation, and conferences for San Diego area; Link to 11 statewide CRCs. Also call Area Agencies on Aging in US or dial 211.
> www.caregivercenter.org, 800-827-1008

Books

Zasler ND, Katz D, & Zafonte R (eds). (2007). *Brain Injury Medicine: Principles and Practice*. Demos Publishers. 2007.

Equipment/Products/Technology Information

AbleData
> Provides database of unbiased information about assistive technology products and rehabilitation equipment available worldwide. Helps locate companies that sell these products.
> www.abledata.com, 800-227-0216

AbleLink Technologies
> Offers products to help with cognitive impairments.
> www.ablelinktech.com

RESNA
> Offers information about assistive technology and tries to connect visitors with experts in their area.
> www.resna.org, 703-524-6686

Alliance for Technology Access
> Network of community-based resource centers. Offers free service to locate and receive information on assistive technology products to promote independence.
> www.ataccess.org, 707-778-3011

Bruce Medical Supply
> General health and medical supplies, some sale items reduced to 35%. Free catalog.
> www.brucemedical.com, 800-225-8446

Center for Assistive Technology (CAT)
> Helps people find, select, and learn to use assistive technology devices and equipment for essential everyday needs: mobility, hearing, speech, and recreation as well as computer, vehicle, and home modifications.
> www.cat.pitt.edu, 412-647-1310

Center for Rehabilitation Technologies (CRT)
> Offers programs to assist people with physical disabilities to increase their independence
> www.helenhayeshospital.org/special_services/crt.htm, 888-70-REHAB (888-707-3422)

Disability Product postcards
> Information about catalogs and many products/equipment in a free monthly packet.
> www.blvd.com/dpp.htm

Cognitive

National Aphasia Association
> Provides information, support and advocacy; sells printed materials. Lists professionals, support groups, and treatment centers by state.
> www.aphasia.org, 800-922-4622

National Center for Learning Disabilities
> Offers information and resources for parents, educators, and students.
> www.ncld.org, 888-575-7373

HANDLE Institute (Holistic Approach to Neurodevelopment and
Learning Efficiency)
Provides clinical services and community information to identify
and treat most neurodevelopmental disorders. Lists numerous
regional practitioners.
www.handle.org, 206-204-6000

Computer Equipment and Software; Internet Games/Exercises

Parrot Software
Software for communication, memory, attention, speech, and
cognitive rehabilitation. Offers free trial of internet programs.
www.parrotsoftware.com, 800-727-7681

HAPPYneuron Brain Fitness
Offers membership with unlimited and ever-changing games for
$10/month.
www.happy-neuron.com, various phone numbers on website.

Thinks.com
Puzzles & Games: Sudoku, Crosswords, Chess, Checkers &
more.
www.thinks.com

Luminosity
Brain training games.
www.lumosity.com

Emotional

Depression and Bipolar Support Alliance (DBSA)
Information, resources, support, products.
www.dbsalliance.org, 800-826-3632
Crisis line number: 800-273-TALK (800-273-8255)

Grief Recovery Online (GROWW)
Chat rooms, message boards, news and information, resource
lists, and support groups for all bereaved people.
www.groww.org

Grief Recovery Helpline
> Answers questions about loss and recovery.
> www.ggcoa.org/r-hl-grief-recovery-helpline.htm, 800-445-4808

Mental Health America (MHA)
> Crisis help and information about disorders, treatments,
> medication, finding a therapist.
> www.nmha.org, 800-969-6642

National Alliance on Mental Illness (NAMI)
> Largest grassroots organization for those who are ill and their
> families, with affiliates in every state and many communities,
> offers information, education, support, advocacy, and helpline.
> www.nami.org, 800-950-NAMI (800-950-6264)

National Clearinghouse for Alcohol and Drug Information (NCADI)
> One-stop resource for information about substance abuse
> prevention and addiction treatment. Confer with information
> specialist, obtain referrals and order publications.
> www.ncadi.samhsa.gov, 800-729-6686

National Institute on Drug Abuse (NIDA)
> Information, materials, and resources for students and young
> adults, parents and teachers, and health professionals.
> www.nida.nih.gov, 301-443-1124

National Institutes of Mental Health (NIMH)
> Research focused on understanding, treating, and preventing
> mental disorders and promoting mental health.
> www.nimh.nih.gov, 866-615-6464

Substance Abuse and Mental Health Services Administration
(SAMHSA)
> Information about national programs, resources, services, and
> finding help.
> www.samhsa.gov, 800-662-HELP (800-662-4357)

Suicide Awareness Voices of Education (SAVE)
> Information, resources, and products for depression and suicide.
> www.save.org, National Suicide Prevention Lifeline 800-273
> TALK (800-273-8255), other numbers on website.

Traditional Medical

General Information

Centers for Disease Control and Prevention (CDC)
> Credible information on all known conditions and diseases as
> well as healthy living and environmental health topics.
> www.cdc.gov, 800-CDC-INFO (800-232-4636)

Mayo Clinic
> Medical services, information on symptoms, diseases and
> conditions, drugs and supplements, and healthy living. Includes
> "Ask a specialist" feature, newsletter.
> www.mayoclinic.com

Medscape
> Provides the latest medical news and access to journal articles on
> lots of topics.
> www.medscape.com

WebMD
> Features include pill identifier, symptom checker, find doctors
> and hospitals, medical news, health A to Z, nutritional
> information, blogs.
> www.webmd.com

Specific Conditions/Treatments

American Tinnitis Association (ATA)
> Information, answers to questions, advocacy, resources,
> newsletter, products, lists professionals and support groups in
> your area.
> www.ata.org, 800-634-8978

Animal-Human Connection
> Many programs and resources, including service animal and pet
> therapy, links, products.
> www.deltasociety.org, 425-679-5500

Canine Companions for Independence
> Trained assistance dogs free of charge.
> www.cci.org, 800-572-BARK (800-572-2275)

Eye Movement and Desensitization and Reprocessing (EMDR) Institute
Technique found to be highly effective for trauma. Includes
information, FAQs, references, locating clinicians.
www.emdr.com, 831-761-1040

Mobility Opportunities Via Education/Experience (MOVE) International
A worldwide program to help people gain independence and
improve mobility; model sites, research, products, FAQs, events.
www.move-international.org, 800-397-MOVE (800-397-6683)

Parents Active for Vision Education (PAVE)
Information, resources, products, blogs, referrals about visual
issues.
www.pavevision.org, 800-728-3988

Vestibular Disorders Association (VEDA)
Information, medical help, publications, products.
www.vestibular.org, 800-837-8428

Products, Devices

Cranial Electrical Stimulation Units (CES) and other healing light and
sound devices.
www.dynamind.com, 888-396-2646
www.sotainstruments.com, 800-224-0242

Light Therapy: many sources of light boxes available online.

Muscle Stimulation/Pain Management Units, including TENS: many
sites listed online.

Stroke Recovery Systems
Rehabilitation device to regain lost limb functionality.
www.neuromove.com, 800-845-1771

Complementary Medicine Resources

General Information

National Center for Complementary and Alternative Medicine
(NCCAM)
Offers research-based information on A to Z treatments and
conditions, FAQs, live online and phone help.
www.nccam.nih.gov, 888-644-6226

Health World Online
> Provides trustworthy information on wellness, healthy living, alternative therapies, body-mind-spirit health; finding practitioners.
> www.healthy.net

Specific Treatments

American Association of Acupuncture & Oriental Medicine (AAAOM)
> Consumer portion offers information, history, referrals, links.
> www.aaaomonline.org, 866-455-7999

American Chiropractic Association
> Patient section offers information, history, links, referrals, FAQs.
> www.amerchiro.org

American Massage Therapy Association
> Consumer section offers information, resources, links, find therapist, FAQs.
> www.amtamassage.org, 877-905-2700

American Osteopathic Association (AOA)
> Holistic medicine; information, links, resources, FAQs.
> www.osteopathic.org; 800-621-1773

American Society of Clinical Hypnosis
> Public site explains uses, myths, offers links, referrals, resources.
> www.asch.net, 630-980-4740

Energy Healing: These methods focus and amplify your life force (Chi)
> to help your body to naturally heal itself; sites offer history, information, practitioners, resources, blog.
> www.quantumtouch.com, 888-424-0041
> www.reiki.com

Feldenkrais Method of Somatic Education:
> Offers information, resources, FAQs, publications.
> www.feldenkrais.com, 800-775-2118

Trager Approach
> History, information, find practitioner, articles.
> www.trager.com

World Wide Online Meditation Center|
    Offers information, instruction on many techniques, resources,
    books, products, FAQs.
    www.meditationcenter.com

Nutrition

General Information

Center for Science in the Public Interest (CSPI)
    Nutrition and health, public safety, and sound science; "Nutrition
    Action" is largest circulation health newsletter in North America.
    www.cspinet.org, 202-332-9110

Harvard School of Public Health, Dept. of Nutrition
    Healthy eating guidelines and tips, recipes, FAQs, dispels myths.
    www.hsph.harvard.edu/nutritionsource

Mayo Clinic Nutrition and Healthy Eating
    Information about healthy eating and cooking, free newsletter.
    www.mayoclinic.com/health/nutrition-and-healthy-
    eating/MY00431

Queensland nutrition website
    Healthy eating, activity, and food safety tips, news, and
    resources.
    www.health.qld.gov.au/healthieryou/food

US Dept. of Agriculture
    Lots of info, guidelines, helps to plan/track health and activity to
    manage weight/eating, resources, links.
    www.mypyramid.gov, 888-7-PYRAMID (888-779-7264)

Also see General Information under Traditional Medical

Physical

General Fitness/Health Information

MyStart!
> Free American Heart Association (AHA) online tool to help
> people make positive lifestyle changes through physical activity
> and better eating.
> www.americanheart.org/presenter.jhtml?identifier=3053103

Disability-Related Fitness/Sports/Recreation

Blaze Sports
> Provides sports training, competitions, summer camps, and other
> recreational opportunities to youth and adults with disabilities;
> current calendar, magazine; memberships available.
> www.blazesports.org, 770-850-8199

Disabled Sports USA
> Nationwide network of community-based chapters that offers
> sports and recreational programs; magazine, equipment
> resources.
> www.dsusa.org, 301-217-0960

Disabled Sports USA Far West
> Offers special events, plus 200+ program days, links, newsletter.
> www.dsusafw.org, 916-722-6447

Disaboom
> An interactive online disability community for people with
> disabilities and their loved ones; offers health-lifestyle
> information, news, groups, blogs.
> www.disaboom.com

National Center on Physical Activity and Disability (NCPAD)
> Comprehensive information on many disabilities/conditions,
> including all aspects of fitness programs; organized by state and
> country, suppliers, references, resources, videos, research;
> nutrition; newsletter; search mechanism; free information
> service. Free "virtual trainer" tips sent by email.
> www.ncpad.org, 800-900-8086

National Sports Center for the Disabled
Offers adaptive recreation clinics and programs in over 20 sports throughout the US, including competitive skiing.
www.nscd.org, 970-726-1540

Re-Creative Resources, Inc.
"Recreating mind, body and spirit" website that lists hundreds of products and providers; links, resources; go to Resources/Links, then Programming for adaptive equipment, leisure activities, crafts, music.
www.recreativeresources.com, 732-340-1210

Specific Activities/Sports/Populations

Active Network
nationwide listing of events in all sports, registration, training logs, nutrition, training and fitness tips, resources, race results, blogs.
www.active.com

Our Ocean Dreams
Aquatic experiences; learn to dive anywhere there's water, nationwide network of divers; online certification courses.
www.ouroceandreams.com, 727-578-3095

Extremity Games
Yearly sports competition for those with limb loss or difference; events include Moto-X, skateboarding, rock climbing, wakeboarding, kayaking, mountain biking, martial arts; blog.
www.extremitygames.com, 586-556-1761

Holden Arboretum, Accessible Gardening/Horticulture Therapy
programs, classes, activities, tours, resources.
www.holdenarb.org, 440-946-4000

Hippotherapy (rehabilitative horseback riding), horticulture therapy; supported employment; attractions include aquarium, rainforest.
www.moodygardens.com/Hope_Therapy, 800-582-4673

National Center for Equine Facilitated Therapy (CEFT)
Offers programs, activities, therapeutic riding.
www.nceft.org, 650-851-2271

Wheelchair Sports, Recreation & Accessible Travel
> Lists 39 web sites that offer a variety of active programs for those with disabilities; links/resources.
> www.usatechguide.org

Equipment (listed by company)
Abilitations
> Specialized equipment for physical and mental development through movement. Products, articles, activity guides.
> www.abilitations.com, 800-850-8602

Access to Recreation, Inc.
> Wide range of indoor and outdoor adaptive equipment and products.
> www.accesstr.com, 800-634-4351

Achievable Concepts
> Australian company selling adapted recreation and sporting equipment products worldwide.
> www.achievableconcepts.com.au

FlagHouse
> A global supplier of over 20,000 physical education, recreation, health care products. Free catalog.
> www.flaghouse.com, 800-793-7900

S&S Worldwide
> Educational, rehab, and therapy products, games and activities. Free catalog.
> www.ssww.com, 800-288-9941

For sport-specific equipment, videos, journals, and books, go to Resources at www.rewiring.org

Social

Brain and Spinal Cord Injury Information and Support Groups
> blog, video library, resources.
> www.brainandspinalcord.org, 800-800-0640

Chat Rooms for survivors
    www.braininjurychat.org
    www.tbichat.org

Chat Rooms for survivors and loved ones, message boards, member
    pages
    www.tbihome.org

Vocational/Community Reentry

Education

Higher Education/Training for People with Disabilities (HEATH)
    Information, including financial assistance, for students with
    disabilities who seek post-secondary education and/or training.
    www.heath.gwu.edu

Employment

Job Accommodation Network (JAN)
    Free consultation, information, and technical support to job
    seekers and employers about opportunities, training, and rights.
    www.jan.wvu.edu, 800-526-7234

Office of Disability Employment Policy (ODEP)
    Information on employment supports; sites for veterans; links;
    resources.
    www.dol.gov/odep, 866-ODEP-DOL (866-633-7365)

Ticket to Work Program:
    For Social Security recipients. Obtain vocational rehabilitation
    services through your state agency and explore work options
    without losing benefits in this federal program. Employment
    regulations, supports, and work incentives; locate forms and
    publications.
    www.socialsecurity.gov/work, 800-772-1213

Traumatic Brain Injury National Resource Center
    Employment resources.
    www.neuro.pmr.vcu.edu/LINKS/employ.htm

Veterans' Employment and Training Service (VETS)
>   Recovery & Employment Assistance Lifelines program (REALifelines) designed to provide a seamless, personalized assistance network for returning injured and wounded service members.
>   www.dol.gov/vets, 866-4-USA-DOL (866-487-2365)

Financial/Legal

David L. Goldin, APC
>   Articles, news, links, free consultation for survivors/loved ones; member of San Diego BIF.
>   www.brain-injuries-law.com, 866-HEADLAW (866-432-3529)

Equal Employment Opportunities Commission (EEOC)
>   General advice about ADA disability claims; how to file; locate local office.
>   www.eeoc.gov, 800-669-4000

National Insurance Consumer Helpline
>   Consumer support for questions and problems relating to insurance.
>   www.cancerandcareers.org/resources/one?resource_id=56278, 800-942-4242

Renter Assistance: Call your state franchise tax board or Volunteer Income Tax Assistance (see below) for application information.

Social Security Administration (SSA)
>   Federal source to learn about, apply, and appeal for SSDI (disability) and SSI; locate forms and publications.
>   www.ssa.gov, 800-772-1213

Veterans' Administration Benefits
>   Information about education, rehabilitation, benefits, FAQs, finding facilities, links; apply online.
>   www.vba.va.gov/VBA, 800-827-1000

Volunteer Income Tax Assistance
>   IRS-sponsored program with volunteers to provide free tax preparation assistance to low income, disabled, and/or military filers.
>   www.vita-volunteers.org

Housing/Medical

HUD-Federal Housing Authority (HA)
> Answers to questions about housing choice vouchers (Section 8), Self Sufficiency Program.
> www.hud.gov/renting, numerous 800 numbers on website

Medicare
> Medicare and Medicaid coverage, prescription plans; apply, appeal; ask questions.
> www.medicare.gov, 800-MEDICARE (800-633-4227)

Rural Information Center
> For those who live in rural areas; information about education, funding sources, health, and starting a business.
> ric.nal.usda.gov, 800-633-7701

Vocational Rehabilitation

Non-Vets: Search online by for your state agency, look under state listings in local phone book (it may be called Agency, Department, Division, or Office), or go to www.socialsecurity.gov/work, 800-772-1213, for "Ticket To Work" information

Veterans with service-connected disabilities: Vocational Rehabilitation and Employment Service (VR&E) provides evaluation, counseling, assistance, and training for vets to prepare for, find, and keep suitable jobs; site lists resources, links, how to apply www.vba.va.gov/bln/vre

References

Chapter 3: Brain Construction and Wiring General Rewiring

Self, Sept., 1997, p. 165.

Stahl, SM (1996). *Essential psychopharmacology*. London: Cambridge University Press.

Stein, D., Brailowsky, S., & Will, B. (1995). *Brain repair*. New York: Oxford University Press.

Chapter 4: Spiritual Rewiring

Barfield, C. (1998). A blend of faith: Native Americans here practice Catholicism while retaining much of their culture. It's called "syncretism." *San Diego Union-Tribune*, Current & Arts section, E-1, Friday, June 12, 1998.

Being Jewish: The hands-on supplement for Jewish Family Education. (1998). David Epstein, Publisher.

Campbell, D. (1998). *Bottom Line/Personal*, January 15, 1998.

Campbell, D. (1997). *The Mozart Effect: Tapping the Power of Music to Heal the Body, Strengthen The Mind, and Unlock the Creative Spirit*. New York: Avon Books.

Cool, Lisa Collier. (1997). Faith & Healing. *American Health*, 47.

Craughwell, T. Ed. (1998). *Every Eye Beholds You: A World Treasury of Prayer*. New York: Book-of-the-Month Club. Pp. xiv-xvii, 11, 13, 14, 17, 21-22, 171-172, 207-208, 225

Dharma Haven Home Page: http://dharma-haven.org/tibetan/meaning-of-om-mani-padme-hung.htm.

Dembling, Sophia. (1998). Mix, match for workout tape that keeps pace. *San Diego Union-Tribune*, Current & Arts section, E-3, Monday, May 25, 1998.

Graham, J. in Dolbee, S. Holy Humor. The San Diego Union-Tribune, Current & Arts section, Religion & Ethics, E-3 3, Friday, June 19, 1998.

Grey, A. The history of art and healing, Healing ourselves with art, How art heals: Mind-body physiology, Art as a healing force. www.artashealing.org.

Peale, N.V. (1997). *The Art of Praying: A Guide to Confident Living*. New York: Prentice-Hall.

Phoenix & Arabeth. (1998). Shamanic origin of the arts. http://www.zapcom.net/phoenix.arabeth/shaman.html. 7/26/98

Williams, G.III. (1996). The healing power of prayer. *McCalls*, 86-89, April 1996.

Chapter 5: Cognitive Rewiring

Abdulla, S. (2001). Drill helps adult dyslexics: Brain imaging is hot on the trail of dyslexia. Science Update. www.nature.com/nsu/010222/010222-5.html

Askenasy, J.J., & Rahmani, L. (1987). Neuropsycho-social rehabilitation of head injury. *American Journal of Physical Medicine*, 66(6), 315.

Ben-Yishay et al. (1987). cited in Wachter J, Fawber H.L., & Scott, M.B. Vocational Evaluation. In M. Ylvisaker & E. Gobble (Eds.). *Community Re-entry for Head Injured Adults* (pp. 260-277). Boston: College-Hill.

Deaton, A. (1991). Rehabilitating cognitive impairments through use of games. In Kreutzer, J & Wehman, P, Eds., *Cognitive Rehabilitation For Persons with Traumatic Brain Injury*. Baltimore, MD: Paul H. Brookes Publishing Co.

Eriksson, P.S., Perfilieva, E., Björk-Eriksson. T., Alborn, A., Nordborg, C., Peterson, D.A. & Gage, F.H. (1998). Neurogenesis in the adult human hippocampus. *Nature Medicine*, 4(11), 1313.

Hamm, RJ; Temple, MD; O'Dell, DM; Pike, BR; Lyeth, BG. (1996). Exposure to environmental complexity promotes recovery of cognitive function after traumatic brain injury. *Journal of Neurotrauma*, 13(1):41-7.

Johnson, DW (1999). Antiaging Strategies: for your body, for your mind. *Bottom Line Health.* 13 (2), 2.

Levin, W. (1991). Computer Applications in Cognitive Rehabilitation. In Kreutzer, J & Wehman, P, Eds., *Cognitive Rehabilitation For Persons with Traumatic Brain Injury.* Baltimore, MD: Paul H. Brookes Publishing Co.

Levine, B., Cabeza, R., McIntosh, A.R., Black S.E., Grady C.L., Stuss D.T. (2002). Functional reorganization of memory after traumatic brain injury: a study with H_2O positron emission tomography. *Journal Neurology Neurosurgery Psychiatry, 73*(2): 111

Najenson, T., Mendelson, L., Schechter, I., David, C., Mintz, N., & Groswasser, Z. (1974). Rehabilitation after severe head injury. *Scandinavian Journal of Rehab. Medicine, 6*, 5.

Namerov, N.S. (1987). Cognitive and behavioral aspects of brain-injury rehabilitation. *Neurologic Clinics, 5*(4), 569.

Parente, R. & Anderson-Parente, JK. (1991). Retraining memory: Theory, evaluation, and applications. In Kreutzer, J & Wehman, P, Eds., *Cognitive Rehabilitation For Persons with Traumatic Brain Injury.* Baltimore, MD: Paul H. Brookes Publishing Co.

Sbordone, R. (1991). Overcoming obstacles in cognitive rehabilitation of persons with severe traumatic brain injury. In Kreutzer, J & Wehman, P, Eds., *Cognitive Rehabilitation For Persons with Traumatic Brain Injury.* Baltimore, MD: Paul H. Brookes Publishing Co.

Stein, D., Brailowsky, S. & Will, B. (1995). *Brain Repair.* London:Oxford University Press.

Vogenthaler, D.R. (1987). Subject review: an overview of head injury: Its consequences and rehabilitation. *Brain Injury, 1*(1), 113.

Chapter 6: Emotional Rewiring

Baser, C. Personal Communication. 11 May 1995.

Baser, C. Personal Communication. 5 December 1997.

Bigler, ED, Blatter, DD, Johnson, SC, Anderson, CV, Russo, AA, Gale, SD, Ryser, DK, MacNamara, SE, Bailey, BJ. (1996). Traumatic brain injury, alcohol and quantitative neuroimaging: preliminary findings. *Brain Injury 10*(3):197-206.

Bolla KL; Funderburk FR; Cadet JL. (2000). Differential effects of cocaine and cocaine alcohol on neurocognitive performance. *Neurology, 54*(12):2285-92.

Cobble, ND, Bontke, CF, Brandstater, ME, & Horn, LJ. (1991). Rehabilitation in brain disorders. 3. Intervention strategies. *Archives of Physical Medicine and Rehabilitation, 72*, S324-S331.

Corrigan, JD, Bogner, JA, Lamb-Hart, GL, & Windisch, E. (1996). Effectiveness of a case management model for treatment of substance abuse following acquired brain injury. Columbus, Ohio: Ohio Valley Center for Head Injury Prevention and Rehabilitation.

Corrigan, JD, Bogner, JA, Mysiw, WJ, Clinchot, D & Fugate, LP. (1997). Systematic bias in outcome studies of persons with traumatic brain injury. *Archives of Physical Medicine and Rehabilitation, 78*(2):132-7.

Corrigan, JD., Lamb-Hart, G. (2004). Substance abuse issues after brain injury. *Living with Brain Injury,* BIAUSA.

Corrigan, JD., Rust, E., Lamb-Hart, GL. (1995). The nature and extent of substance abuse problems in persons with traumatic brain injury. *Journal of Head Trauma Rehabilitation, 10*(3): 29-46.

Hendryx, PM. (1989). Psychosocial changes perceived by closed head-injured adults and their families. *Archives of Physical Medicine and Rehabilitation, 70*: 526-530.

Isenhart, Mary Alice. Personal communication. 9-22-94.

Kay, T. (1986). *Minor head injury: An introduction for professionals.*, Southboro, MA: National Head Injury Foundation.

Kendler, K, Aggen, S, Tambs, K, & Reichborn-Kjennerud, T. (2006). Illicit psychoactive substance use, abuse and dependence in a population-based sample of Norwegian twins. *Psycholgical Medicine, 36*(7):955-962.

Khalsa, JH, Genser, S, Francis, H, Martin, B. (2002). Clinical consequences of marijuana. *J Clin Pharmacol. 42*(11 Suppl): 75-105

Koob, GF. (2006). Alcohol dependence: The importance of neurobiology to treatment. *Medscape Psychiatry & Mental Health, 11*(2).

Kreutzer, JS, Witol, AD, Sander, AM, Cifu, DX, Marwitz, JH, Delmonico, R. (1996). A prospective longitudinal multicenter analysis of alcohol use patterns among persons with traumatic brain injury. *Journal of Head Trauma Rehabilitation, 11*(5): 58-69.

Kreutzer, J, Marwitz, JH, Witol, AD, (1995). Interrelationships between crime, substance abuse, and aggressive behaviours among persons with traumatic brain injury. *Brain Injury*, *9*(8), 757-68.

Kubler-Ross, E. (1969). *On death and dying.* New York: Macmillan.

Little, KY, Krolewski DM, Zhnag L, Cassin BJ. (2003). Loss of striatal vesicular monamine transporter protein in human cocaine users. *Am. Jrnl of Psychiatry, 160*(1):47-55.

Lovinger, DP. (1999). The role of serotonin in alcohol's effects on the brain. *Current Separations, 18*(1): 23-28.

Mameli-Engvall, M; Evrard, A; Pons, S; Maskos, U; Svensson, T; Changeux, JP; Faure, P. (2006). Hierarchical control of dopamine neuron-firing patterns by nicotinic receptors. *Neuron.* June 15, 2006.

National Institute on Drug Abuse (NIDA), National Institutes of Health (NIH). (2006). NIDA Infofacts: Crack and cocaine. www.drugabuse.gov/Infofacts/cocaine.html.

National Institute on Drug Abuse (NIDA), National Institutes of Health (NIH). (2004). Research Report: Cocaine Abuse and Addiction. Pub. # 99-4342. Revised November 2004.

Prigatano, GP. (1987). Neuropsychological deficits, personality variables, and outcome. In M. Ylvisaker & E. Gobble, Eds. *Community Re-Entry for Head Injured Adults.* Boston: College Hill.

RTC-Research & Training Ctr. on Community Integration of Individuals with TBI. (2000). Consumer Report # 6: Coping with Substance Abuse After TBI, Mt. Sinai School of Med.

RTC-Research & Training Ctr. on Community Integration of Individuals with TBI. (1999). *Consumer Report # 4*: Coping with Post-TBI Emotional Distress. Mt. Sinai School of Med.

Tanner, DC. (1984). *Aphasia: The family's guide to the psychology of loss, grief, and adjustment.* Tulsa: Modern Education Corporation.

Thomsen, IV. (1984). Late outcomes of very severe blunt head trauma: A 10-15 year second follow-up. *Journal of Neurology, Neurosurgery, and Psychiatry, 47*, 260-268.

To, SE. (2006). Alcoholism and pathways to recovery: New survey results on views and treatment options. *Medscape General Medicine 8*(1):2.

United States Congress, Office of Technology Assessment. (1993). Biological components of substance abuse and addiction. OTA-BP-BBS-117. Washington, DC: US Government Printing Office. ISBN: 0-16-042096-2. www.norml.org/research/aa/aaota-cont.html.

University of Washington Department of Rehabilitation Medicine. (1998). New research sheds light on alcohol use after brain injury. *Brain Injury Rehabilitation Update.* 11-21-98. http://weber.u.washington.edu/~rehab/bi/update/9-1alcohol.html.

Zickler, P. (2003). Cocaine's effect on blood components may be linked to heart attack and stroke. *NIDA Notes, 17*(6). www.drugabuse.gov/NIDA_notes

Zickler, P. (2004). Cocaine may compromise immune system, increase risk of infection. *NIDA Notes, 18*(6). www.drugabuse.gov/NIDA_notes

Chapter 7: Body-Mind Rewiring

Baser, C. (1998). Personal communication.

Bennington, K. (1997). Eye movement desensitization and reprocessing. Unpublished paper and personal communication.

Dupler, J. (1998). Neurofeedback as an alternative treatment for head injury. Rewiring.org

Gardner, D. (1992). When to push pills: The role of medication treatment in TBI. *Total Quality Newsletter, 1*(2). Neurocare, Inc.

Gizzi, M. (1995). The efficacy of vestibular rehabilitation for patients with head trauma. *The Journal of Head Trauma Rehabilitation. 10*(6):60.

Health Confidential. (1996). (Interview of George Brainerd) Light therapy to beat: Heart disease, insomnia, depression, and more. *Health Confidential, 5.*

Klawansky S, Yeung A, Berkey C, Shah N, Phan H, Chalmer, TC. (1995). Meta-analysis of randomized controlled trials of cranial electrostimulation. Efficacy in treating selected psychological and physiological conditions. *Journal of Nervous and Mental Disorders. 183*(7):478-84.

Kosses, R. (2004). Two types of E-Stim. *Rehab Management.* www.rehabpub.com/features/82004/3.asp

La Fazio, J. (1997). In Vincent, K. Creativity as a healing tool. *Brain Injury Press 1.*

Miller, E. (2008). Music therapy & biofeedback. Expressive Therapy Concepts, Article 1. www.expressivetherapy.org/bioart.html.

Moldover, JE, Goldberg, KB, Prout, MF. (2004). Depression after traumatic brain injury: A review of evidence for clinical hetereogeneity. *Neuropsychol Rev. 14*(3):143-54.

National Center for Equine-Facilitated Therapy. (1997). http://204.188.13.36/hippo/. 11-7-97.

Robinson, R. (1992). EMDR...A breakthrough in therapy. *Bulletin of the Australian Psychological Society.* April 1992.

Seel, RT, Kreutzer, JS, Rosenthal, M, Hammond, FM, Corrigan, JD, & Black, K. (2003). Depression after traumatic brain injury: A National Institute on Disability and Rehabilitation Research Model Systems multicenter investigation. *Arch Phys Med Rehabil. 84*(2):177-84.

.Shumway-Cook, A. Vestibular Rehabilitation. www.vestibular.org/rehab.html.

Tufts University Diet & Nutrition Letter. (1994). Shedding dietary light on Seasonal Affective Disorder. Vol. 12(1).

Voelker, R. (1995). Puppy love can be therapeutic, too. *JAMA 274*(24):1897.

Weil, A. (1997). EMDR for traumatic memories. *Self Healing, 2.*

Chapter 8: Mind–Body-Spirit Rewiring

Altman, L. (1997) Study on using magnets to treat pain surprises skeptics. *New York Times.* December 9, 1997.

American Chiropractic Association, (1990). Chiropractic offers long-term headache relief. www.amerchiro.org/consumer/ha-study.htm 8/27/98

Bezilla, T. (1997). Traditional osteopathy as a model for holistic medicine. *Magazine of the AHMA.* Spring, 1997. ahmaholistic.com/journal2articles97/osteopathy.html.

Caldecott, H. (1996). The promise of energy healing. *SELF,* November 1996, pp.161-168, 173-174.

Dannheisser, I & Edwards, P. (1998). *Homeopathy: An illustrated guide.* Boston: Element Books.

Feely, R. Cranial osteopathy FAQ. RHEMA Medical Associates Limited www.rhemamed.com/cranfaq.htm

Foley, D. (2004). Picking up good vibrations. *Prevention.* October 2004. pp. 172-173, 202.

Gach, M. (1997). Acupressure: How to use it to relieve common ailments. *BottomLine Health.* February 1997. pp. 5-6.

Gardner, JG. (2000) *A healer's voice.* St. Paul, MN: Tree of Life Press.

Heel, Inc. AMA journal publishes positive study of homeopathic medication for vertigo. www.naturalhealthvillage.com/newsletter/HL980825.htm.

Horton, CT. Getting a grip with reflexology. www.doubleclickd.com/reflexology.html

International Center for Reiki Training. www.reiki.org.

Jahnke, R. (1997). Secrets of self-healing from chinese medicine. *Bottom Line Health,* September 1997, pp. 3-4

Jin Shin Jyutsu, Inc. www.Jinshinjyutsu

Kaplan, G. (1998). Acupuncture really works. *Bottom Line Health.* March 1998, pp. 11-12.

La Voie, A. (1997). Magnets may help battle depression. Health World Online. *American Journal of Psychiatry. 154*:1752-56.

Lewith, G. Modern acupuncture methods. HealthWorld Online. www.healthy.net/library/books/modacu/mod2.HTM

Mac Dorman, C. (1996). Acupuncture: America's latest healing miracle: Effective treatment for brain injury. Rewiring.org.

Mahoney, S. (2004). May the force be with you. *Prevention.* pp. 170-171, 200.

Moline, J. Massage is good medicine. www2.spafinders.com/magazine_f_massage.html.

Moyers, B. (1993). *Healing and the Mind.* New York: Doubleday

Namikoshi, T. (1981). *The complete book of shiatsu therapy.* Tokyo: Japan Publications, Inc.

Poirot, C. (1998). Magnets' attraction? Pain relief for athletes. Health World Online. Today's Healthy News from *Fort Worth Star-Telegram.* 8/28/98

Redwood, D. Meditation and relaxation. Health World Online. pp. 1-9 http://205.180.229.2/library/articles/DanRedwood//meditat.htm

Rondberg, T. (1996). *Chiropractic first.* San Diego: Chiropractic Journal.

Tappan, F. (1980). *Healing massage techniques. A study of Eastern and Western methods.* Reston, VA: Reston Publishing Co.

Tsuei, J. (1996). Scientific evidence in support of acupuncture and meridian theory. *Institute of Electrical and Electronics Engineers, Engineering in Medicine and Biology Magazine, 15* (3).

Wiancko, K. (1995). Magnetotherapy: Ancient wisdom, modern use. *Health Naturally.* April/May 1995. p. 29.

Williams, T. (1996). The complete illustrated guide to Chinese medicine: A comprehensive system for health and fitness. Boston: Element.

Chapter 9: Nutritional Rewiring

Broadhurst, CL, Cunnane, SC, Crawford, MA. (1998). Rift Valley lake fish and shellfish provided brain-specific nutrition for early Homo. *British Journal of Nutrition, 79*(1).

Friedman School of Nutrition Science and Policy.(2004). And to all a good night: How sleep deprivation may lead to chronic disease. Special Supplement to the Tufts University Health and Nutrition Letter. October 2004

Harvard School of Public Health. Nicotine level increase. *Web MD Magazine*, Nov-Dec., 2007.

Jegalian, K. (1998). Smoking out the cause of addiction: Genetic coding may affect how hard it is to quit. *San Diego Union-Tribune*, Current & Arts Section, pp. 1, 3. Monday, August 17, 1998.

Johnson, DW (1999). Antiaging Strategies: For your body, for your mind. *Bottom Line Health, 13*(2):2.

Kotulak, R. (1998). Skimping on sleep may make you fat, clumsy, and haggard. *San Diego Union-Tribune*, (from *Chicago Tribune*), pp. A25, 26, June 14, 1998.

Margen, S. and the Editors of the University of California at Berkeley Wellness Letter. (1992). *The wellness encyclopedia of food and nutrition*. New York: Rebus.

Mayo Clinic Staff. Snack attack: Know what foods to choose when hunger strikes. www.mayoclinic.com/invoke.cfm?id=HQ01396, www.mypyramid.gov.

Roan, S. (2008). How lack of sleep may be bad for the brain. *Los Angeles Times*, Health, 3-24-08

Scripps Clinic and Research Foundation, division of chest, critical care medicine, sleep disorders clinic. (1989). Learning how to sleep better as you age. *Patient Care*. April 30, 1989.

Stein, D., Brailowsky, S, and Will, B. (1995). *Brain Repair*. New York: Oxford University Press.

Chapter 10: Physical Rewiring

Bray, LJ, Carlson, F, Humphrey, R, Mastrelli, J, & Valso, A. (1987). Physical Rehabilitation. In M. Ylvisaker & E. Gobble (Eds.), *Community Re-Entry for Head Injured Adults*. Boston: College-Hill.

Cohadon, F., Richter, E., Reglade, C., Dartigues, JF. (1988). Recovery of motor function after severe traumatic coma. *Scandinavian Journal of Rehabilitation Medicine Supplement. 17*:75-85.

Dobkin, BH. (2000). Functional rewiring of brain and spinal cord after injury: The three Rs of neural repair and technological rehabilitation. *Current Opinion in Neurology, 13*:655-659.

Dordel, HJ. (1989). Intensive mobility training as a means of late rehabilitation after brain injury. *Adapted Physical Activity Quarterly. 6*:176-187.

Durstine, J.L., Painter, P., Franklin, B.A., Morgan, D., Pitetti, K.H., & Roberts S.O. http://www.ingentaconnect.com/content/adis/smd/2000/00000030/000 00003/art00005 - aff_6(2000). Physical activity for the chronically ill and disabled. *Sports Medicine, Supplement 30*(3):207-219

Evans, K. (1997). How to gong your own qi. *Health*, March 1997. p. 102.

Gordon, W., Sliwinski, M., Echo, J., McLoughlin, M., Sheerer, M., Meili, T. (1998). The benefits of exercise in individuals with traumatic brain injury: A retrospective study. *Journl of Head Trauma Rehab 13*(4):58-67.

Griffith, E. (1983). Spasticity. In Rosenthal, M. *Rehabilitation of the head injured adult,* Philadelphia: FA Davis.

Isenhart, MA. (1992). Personal communication.

Kottke, FJ., (1980). From reflex to skill: the training of coordination. *Archives of Physical Medicine and Rehabilitation, 61*:551-561.

LeMay, M. (2003). The stretch cure. *Bottom Line Health, 17*(12):13-14.

Liu, L. (1997). PulseMind/Body. *American Health, 18.*

Mercer, L. & Boch, M. (1983). Residual sensorimotor deficits in the adult head-injured patient. *Physical Therapy, 63*(12):1988-1991.

Moline, J. (1998). Tai chi. *Spafinder magazine, 1,*.www2.spafinders.com/magazine_f_taichi.html 8/27/98

Moyers, B. (1993). *Healing and the Mind*. New York: Doubleday.

National Center for Chronic Disease Prevention and Health Promotion. (1996). Physical activity and health: A report of the surgeon general; persons with disabilities. www.cdc.gov/nccdphp/sgr/disab.htm. 9/24/2004

Neporent, L. & Schlosberg, S. (1996). *Fitness for Dummies*. New York: For Dummies.

Rinehart, MA. (1983). Considerations for functional training in adults after head injury. *Physical Therapy 63*(12):1975-1982.

Roach, M. (1997). My quest for qi. *Health*, 97, March 1997.

Rogers, R. (1990). In Brady, S. Brain gym helps those on mend from severe neurological disorders. *North County Times*, B-1, March 3, 1998.

Wildman, F. (1986). The Feldenkrais method: Clinical applications. *Physical Therapy Forum. V*(8):3-4

Yogabasics.com.Types of yoga. www.yogabasics.com/yoga/YogaStyles.html.

Chapter 11: Social Rewiring

Baser, C. Personal communications, 10-22-98, 1-21-99.

Blais MC & Boisvert JM. (2007). Psychological adjustment and marital satisfaction following head injury: Which critical personal characteristics should both partners develop? *Brain Injury, 21*(4):357-72.

Burke, WH. (editor) (1997). Head injury rehabilitation: Developing social skills, rev. ed. HDI Series #9. Houston: HDI Publishers.

Burton, LA, Leahy, DM, & Volpe, B. (2003). Traumatic brain injury brief outcome interview. (Abstract) *Applied Neuropsychol, 10*(3):145-152.

Corrigan, JD, Rust, E, &Lamb-Hart, G. (1995). The nature and extent of substance abuse problems in persons with traumatic brain injury. *Journal of Head Trauma Rehabilitation, 10*(3):29-46.

Corrigan, JD, Bogner, JA, Mysiw, WJ, Clinchot, D, & Fugate, L. (2001). Life satisfaction after traumatic brain injury. *Journal of Head Trauma Rehabilitation, 16*(6):543-55.

Dawson, DR; & Chipman, M. (1995). The disablement experienced by traumatically brain-injured adults living in the community. *Brain Injury, 9*(4):339-53.

Dolberg, O, Klag, E, Gross, Y, & Schreiber S. (2002). Relief of serotonin selective reuptake inhibitor induced sexual dysfunction with low-dose mianserin in patients with traumatic brain injury. *Psychopharmacology, 161*(4):404-407.

Gisi, TM & D'Amato, RC. (2000). What factors should be considered in rehabilitation: Are anger, social desirability, and forgiveness related in adults with traumatic brain injuries? *Intl Journal Neurosci 105*(1-4):121-33.

Goldstein, I. (1996).New strategies for overcoming impotence. *Health Confidential*, December 1996.

Hein, J. TBI Group Meetings notes: 1997, 1998 (6-18-98)

Hoofien, D, Gilboa, A, Vakil, E, & Donovick, PJ. (2001). Traumatic brain injury (TBI) 10-20 years later: A comprehensive outcome study of psychiatric symptomatology, cognitive abilities and psychosocial functioning. *Brain Injury 15*(3):189-209.

Isenhart, MaryAlice. Personal communication, 1991-92

Kreuter, M, Sullivan, M, Dahliof, AG, & Siosteen, A. (1998). Partner relationships, functioning, mood and global quality of life in persons with spinal cord injury and traumatic brain injury. *Spinal Cord 36*(4):252-61.

Kreutzer, J., Marwitz, JH., & Witol, AD. (1995). Interrelationships between crime, substance abuse, and aggressive behaviours among persons with traumatic brain injury. *Brain Injury, 9*(8):757.

Mamelak, M. (2000). The motor vehicle collision injury syndrome. *Neuropsychiatry Neuropsychology Behavioral Neurol, 13*(2):125-35.

Namerov, N. (1987). Cognitive and behavioral aspects of brain-injury rehabilitation. *Neurologic Clinics, 5*(4):569-583.

Powell, J, Heslin, J, & Greenwood, R. (2002). Community-based rehabilitation after severe traumatic brain injury: A randomized controlled trial. *Journal of Neurology, Neurosurgery, and Psychiatry, 72*(2):193-202.

Prigatano, GP. (1987). Neuropsychological deficits, personality variables, and outcome. In Ylvisaker, M & Gobble, E. Eds *Community re-entry for head injured adults*, Boston: College Hill.

Sandel, ME, Williams, KS, Dellapietra, L, & Derogatis, LR. (1996). Sexual functioning following traumatic brain injury. *Brain Injury, 10*(10):719.

Sobel, D & Ornstein, R. (1998). Friends can be good medicine. *Mind/Body Health Newsletter, VII*(1):3.

Stein, D., Brailowsky, S. & Will, B. (1995). *Brain repair*. London: Oxford University Press.

Tate, RL, Fenelon, B, Manning, ML, & Hunter, M. (1991). Patterns of neuropsychological impairment after severe blunt head injury. *The Journal of Nervous and Mental Disease, 179*(3):117-126.

Thomsen, IV. (1992). Late psychological outcome in severe traumatic brain injury. Preliminary results of a third follow-up study after 20 years. *Scand Journal of Rehabilitation Medicine Supplement 26*:142-52.

Wood Rl & Rutterford NA. (2006). Psychosocial adjustment 17 years after severe brain injury. *Journal of Neurosurg Psychiatry, 77*(1):71-3.

Wood, RL, Yurdakul, LK, (1997). Change in relationship status following brain injury. *Brain Injury,* *1*(7):491.

Ylvisaker, MS. (1988). *Head injury rehabilitation: Management of communication and language deficits.* HDI Series #20, Houston: HDI Publishers.

Ylvisaker, MS. (1997). *Management of communication and language deficits, rev. ed.* HDI Series #20, Houston: HDI Publishers.

Zasler, N.D. (1992). Neuromedical diagnosis and management of post-concussive disorders. *Physical Medicine and Rehabilitation: State of the Art Reviews, 6*(1).

Zasler, ND, & Horn, LJ. (1990). Rehabilitative management of sexual dysfunction. *Journal of Head Trauma Rehabilitation, 5*(2):14.

Zasler, N.D., & Kreutzer, J. (1991). Family and sexuality after traumatic brain injury. In Williams, J. & Kay, T., Eds. *Head injury: A family matter.* Baltimore, MD: Paul H Brookes

Chapter 12: Vocational Rewiring

Abrams, S. Social Security disability benefits. http://205.188.218.81/sheriabrams/page2/htm.

Braverrman, SE, Spector, J, Warden, DL,Wilson, BC, Ellis, TE, Bamdad, MJ, & Salazar, AM. (1999). A multidisciplinary TBI inpatient rehabilitation programme for active duty service members as part of a randomized clinical trial. *Brain Injury, 13*(6):405-15

Department of Labor, Office of Disability Employment Policy. (2005). Supported employment. p. 1-3; www.dol.gov/odep/archives/fact/supportd.htm 1/5/2005

Dolen, C. Use of community services by adult head injury survivors in San Diego County, California. Thesis, Summer 1991.

Haffey, W.J., & Lewis, F.D. (1989). Rehabilitation outcomes following traumatic brain injury. *Physical Medicine and Rehabilitation: State of the Art Reviews, 3*(1):203-218.

High, WM, Gordon, WA, Lehmkuhl, LD, Newton, CN, Vandergood, D, Thoi, L, & Courtney, L. (1995). Productivity and service utilization following traumatic brain injury: Results of a survey by the RSA regional TBI centers. *Journal of Head Trauma Rehabilitation, 10*(4):64-80.

Hoofien, D, Gilboa, A, Vakil, E, & Donovick, P. (2001). Traumatic brain injury (TBI) 10-20 years later: A comprehensive outcome study of psychiatric symptomatology, cognitive abilities and psychosocial functioning. *Brain Injury, 15*(3):189-209.

Levack, W, McPherson, K, & McNaughton, H. (2004). Success in the workplace following traumatic brain injury: Are we evaluating what is most important? *Disabil Rehabil, 26*(5):290-8.

Murrey, GJ & Starzinski, D. (2004). An inpatient neurobehavioural rehabilitation programme for persons with traumatic brain injury: Overview of outcome data for the Minnesota Neurorehabilitation Hospital. *Brain Injury, 18*(6):519-31

National Institute on Disability and Rehabilitation Research Office of Special Education and Rehabilitative Services, Dept. of Education. Washington, D.C. (1994). Rehab brief: community integration of individuals with traumatic brain injury. *Bringing Research Into Effective Focus, XVI*(8). ISSN: 0732-2623. www.cais.net/naric/rehab_b/rb-16-8.html. 04/28/97.

Oddy, M., Coughlan, T., Tyerman, A., & Jenkins, D. (1985). Social adjustment after closed head injury: A further follow-up seven years after injury. *Journal of Neurology, Neurosurgery, and Psychiatry, 48*:564-8.

Prigatano, GP. (1987). Neuropsychological deficits, personality variables, and outcome. In Ylvisaker, M., & Gobble, E., Eds. *Community re-entry for head-injured adults.* Boston: College Hill.

Prigatano, G. (1995). 1994 Sheldon Berrol, MD, Senior Lectureship: The problem of lost normality after brain injury. *Journal of Head Trauma Rehabilitation, 10*(3):87-95.

Social Security Online. (2006). Electronic Leaflets: Working while disabled — How we can help? SSA Publication No. 05-10095.

Social Security Online. The Work Site. Ticket to work program questions and answers. www.socialsecurity.gov/work/ResourcesToolkit/legis

Wagner, A, Hammond, F, Sasser, H, & Wiercisiewski, D. (2002). Return to productive activity after traumatic brain injury: Relationship with measures of disability, handicap, and community integration. *Archives of Physical Medicine and Rehabilitation, 83*(1):107-114.

Webb, C, Wrigley, M, Yoels, W, & Fine P. (1995). Explaining quality of life for persons with traumatic brain injuries 2 years after injury. *Archives of Physical Medicine and Rehabilitation, 76*(12):1113-9.

Wehman, P, Kregel, J, Keyser-Marcus, L, Sherron-Targett, P, Campbell, L, West, M, & Cifu, DX. (2003). Supported employment for persons with traumatic brain injury: A preliminary investigation of long-term follow-up costs and program efficiency. *Archives of Physical Medicine and Rehabilitation, 84*(2):192-6.

Wehman, P, Sherron, P, Kregel, J, Kreutzer, J, Tran, S, & Cifu, D. (1993). Return to work for persons following severe traumatic brain injury: Supported employment outcomes after five years. *Am Journal Physical Medicine and Rehabilitation, 72*(6):355-63

West, M. (1995). Aspects of the workplace and return to work for persons with brain injury in supported employment. *Brain Injury, 9*(3):301-13.

West, M. (2001). The changing landscape of return to work: Implications for Supplemental Security Income and Social Security Disability Insurance beneficiaries with TBI. *Brain Injury Source, 5*(1):24-27.

Index

About the Author

Following her brain injury from a 1976 auto accident in a Minnesota snowstorm, Carolyn E. Dolen received the prognosis, "suicide or psych ward." Befitting her feisty personality, she defied that prediction and within twenty years of her trauma earned two master's degrees with high honors, cycled from San Francisco to Santa Barbara in four days and San Diego to Cabo San Lucas in 13 days, and learned to board and kayak surf. Now she defies the concept of "aging" by competing in triathlons and seeking new adventures.

Carolyn's climb up the recovery mountain required rehabilitation in virtually all areas of life, including mental, emotional, physical, vocational, and social domains. (As current friends can attest, she's still working on this last area.) Her *Rewiring* books describe the path others can follow to recover from brain injury.

Carolyn has appeared in print over 100 times, in both authored and edited pieces. Previous publications include columns in the San Diego Brain Injury Foundation newsletter and health/fitness pieces. She also presented at a national ataxia conference and chaired the 1991 San Diego Disability Awareness Week Network (DAWN) activities that received commendation letters and extensive media coverage.

Professionally, she's taught language arts, math, special education, physical education, and health in the Midwest and California to students who range in age from three to forty-three. Currently, Carolyn coaches a stroke survivor at the YMCA and substitutes for teachers in a variety of adult education courses for Ventura Unified School District.

Besides spreading the word about *Rewiring,* this author-athlete works to improve her surfing and triathlon skills. She qualified for the 2009 Team USA in the sprint triathlon and plans to place even higher in the future. To balance body, mind, and spirit, Carolyn bicycles, runs, swims, weight-trains, practices yoga, competes in various races, sings with the Master Chorale of Ventura County, greets visitors at St. Paul's Episcopal Church, and volunteers at numerous athletic and performing arts events. Obviously, this rewired survivor doesn't "do" idleness!

You, too, can thrive — "Just Do It!"